Chemicals for Animal Health Control

Chemicals for Animal Health Control

George C. Brander

Taylor & Francis
London and Philadelphia
1986

UK   Taylor & Francis Ltd, 4 John St., London WC1N 2ET

USA   Taylor & Francis Inc., 242 Cherry St., Philadelphia,
PA 19106–1906

Copyright © G. C. Brander 1986

British Library Cataloguing in Publication Data

Brander, George C.
   Chemicals for animal health control.
   1. Veterinary public health
   I. Title
   636.089'444   SF740

   ISBN 0-85066-358-X
   ISBN 0-85066-311-1 Pbk

**Library of Congress Cataloging in Publication Data
is available**

Typeset by Alresford Typesetting and Design,
Alresford, Hants.
Printed in Great Britain by Taylor & Francis (Printers) Ltd,
Basingstoke, Hants.

Contents

Preface

Great advances have been made in the last thirty years in the development of new chemicals for the treatment and prevention of disease in human beings and animals. At the same time, too, many new insecticides and fungicides have been introduced for farm use for the control of parasites and other infestations present on farm crops and in tree plantations. These developments have strained to the limits the farmer's understanding of both the relative merits of new chemicals and their relevance to his particular problems.

The aim of this book is to discuss the impact of new methods of disease control in animals and to consider many of the fields of therapy which have become important to the farmer if he is to establish a healthy farm unit. A chapter has been included which compares and contrasts the different problems associated with therapy in animals and human beings. This can be important, as so many bacteria and some viruses attack both man and animals. Because of the economic importance of large farm units and the influence they can exert on the environment, it is important that all who work with animals should be aware of the therapy necessary to prevent the appearance of overt disease in an animal population.

The first four chapters are devoted to considering the changes that have taken place in animal therapy over the years, both to counter disease in animals and to prevent the possibility of infection spreading from animals to the human population. The significance of epidemiological studies in the design of preventive programmes for disease control is outlined. In Chapter 4 some of the different techniques which are used for the administration of drugs to animals are described, and these are contrasted with the relatively straightforward method of administration of drugs in the day-to-day treatment of human patients.

Major areas of disease therapy where specific drugs are used are described in detail, with descriptions of the chemical structures used and their effect both on the pathogens and on the animals undergoing treatment. The areas selected for description are: antibiotics and antibacterials, anthelmintics, pesticides, coccidiostats and other antiprotozoal agents, growth promoters and hormones. In each case the more important chemicals for animal use are described, but as the use and approval of chemicals may vary from country to country it is not possible for the lists always to be comprehensive.

A chapter on the legal control of drugs for animals describes the legislation enacted in the United Kingdom, USA and Europe. A final chapter considers the future of drug development and how it will involve genetic engineering techniques and the development of monoclonal antibodies. The information has been provided in a form that will be of value to all those involved in animal production, and also those associated with the development and application of new drugs.

I would like to thank Mrs Sylvia Osborne and Miss Janet Wheeler for the assistance they gave me in preparing the manuscript, and Dr David Wishart for his advice on the chapter on hormones. Mr R. Cullen, Mr M. Matthewson, and Dr D. Rowlands of Coopers Animal Health were of great assistance in the selection and supply of the photographs used to illustrate the chapters on anthelmintics and pesticides.

Thanks are also due to ICI plc for Figures 1.1, 1.2 and 1.3, to Syntex Agribusiness for Figure 4.4, to J. Buswell, Beecham Pharmaceuticals for Figures 5.1 (*a*)–(*e*) and to Coopers Animal Health for Figures 6.1–6.3 and Figures 7.1–7.16.

George Brander
March 1986

1. Early treatments for the control of disease

Introduction

In planning for the immediate post-war period, that is, the early 1950s, a number of international organizations were formed which would be responsible to the United Nations to ensure that scientific advances would be rapidly applied throughout the world. Two of these impinge on both medicine and agriculture: the World Health Organization (WHO) and the Food and Agriculture Organization (FAO).

The World Health Organization was established to ensure that 'positive' health would become available to the populations of the whole world and there would be "complete physical, mental and social well-being". The Food and Agriculture Organization, for its part, was to be responsible for ensuring that adequate food would be grown for consumption by both the human population and the food animals, and that animal disease would be controlled wherever possible. These concepts were ambitious ones and difficult to put into practice throughout the world as the socio-economic levels of the populations varied from country to country.

It was not at the time fully appreciated that the success of any disease control scheme, whether for human or animal disease, depended on its acceptance by the political leaders of each individual country. Experience has shown that disease control in both animal and human populations can only be continually successful where political stability exists. In addition, the population of a country must have an understanding of the methods that have to be used to produce economically effective crops and also should be aware of the significance of the animal diseases that have to be controlled if animal products are to form a significant part of the diet.

Early veterinary treatment

Before 1945, chemicals and extracts of plants had been used for animal treatment over many centuries and their use usually paralleled the use of similar drugs in human treatment.

In the fourth century AD, Publius Vegetius Renatus compiled a work on the diseases of horses and mules which is known as *Mulomedicina* (Toynbee, 1973). His comments could mirror those recorded by veterinary surgeons ever since as they deplore the unthinking use of drugs by the layman. He expresses his worry that so much of animal treatment is not soundly based, and that not enough attention is paid to the signs of disease and methods of diagnosis. He also is at pains to emphasize that veterinary treatment is not a lowly art and that the veterinarian should not consider himself inferior to the physician. To justify this he refers to the economic value of horses and their noble virtues, and to emphasize the importance and difficulties of veterinary studies points out that "the animal cannot speak for itself whereas a man can describe his symptoms".

In Roman times the treatment of horses involved blood-letting and purging applied in a similar manner to human treatment. The care of the feet too was considered important; the hoof was pared and a special ointment containing tar, wormwood, garlic, pig's fat, old oil and vinegar was applied. In the 1930s when horse transport was still much used, the care of the foot was a major part of veterinary training and many of the dressings still contained tar and oil.

The Romans treated their sheep for parasitic mange by the application of a mixture of the juice of boiled lupins, dregs of old wine and olive lees—this mixture was applied three days after shearing. After treatment the sheep were bathed in the sea or in a salt solution. This too was still practised in the 1930s. Skin lesions were treated by scraping the skin and then applying hemlock juice which had been salted and stored in pots in a dung heap for a whole year. Ground sulphur and liquid pitch boiled over a low fire were also considered efficacious. Retained foetal membranes in domestic animals were treated by the application of liquid wax placed direct into the vagina.

Many of the treatments given to animals during the 1920s and 30s, particularly by farmers who did not use veterinary advice, were as crude by present-day standards as those applied in the fourth century AD. Tar, various oils, irritant chemicals such as cantharides (extract of Spanish fly) and salts of mercury, were applied to the skin. Turpentine, large quantities of magnesium salts, and beers such as stout were poured in copious quantities down the throats of sick animals, when a positive diagnosis could not be made.

Disease-specific drugs were rare in veterinary medicine and treatment often consisted of using chemicals which were potentially very toxic. Lead arsenate, nicotine, copper sulphate and carbon tetrachloride were all given by mouth for the control of helminth infestations in cattle and sheep, although none of them were very specific in action or entirely safe. Cattle and sheep were dipped in mixtures of arsenic and sulphur, and phenols and turpentine were injected into the windpipes of cattle to try to control lungworm infestation. Despite the use of such dangerous drugs, fatalities were not as high as might be expected as considerable skill was developed in their use.

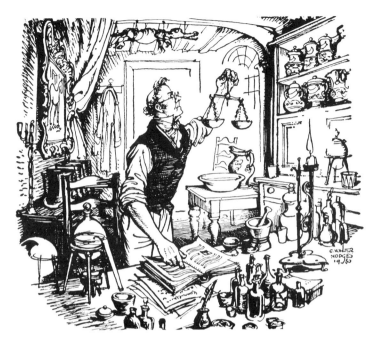

COSTIVENESS
IN CATTLE

Take Linseed, bruised, four ounces;
Tobacco, one ounce;
Common Salt, one handful;
Treacle, four ounces;
Boil the first two articles in three quarts of water; Strain through a linen cloth, and add
remainder. When new-milk warm inject it up the anus.

Figure 1.1.   An old recipe for treating costiveness in cattle.

A crucial balance had to be established between the chances of success of the therapy and the economic value of the animals. Many horses are still cauterized—an irritant liquid or ointment is applied to the skin—or even fired in the effort to speed up recovery from painful damaged tendons.

Figures 1, 2 and 3 illustrate and describe prescriptions which were used in animal medicine in the nineteenth century.

Schwabe (1978) gives a fascinating picture of the development of animal management systems from the days of the Egyptians and Greeks to modern times. Many of the disease problems described by the ancient Egyptians and

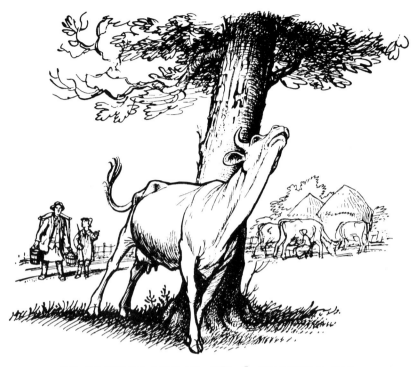

LICE IN CATTLE

Take Hog's Lard, two pounds; Spirit of turpentine, half a pint; Oil of Vitriol one ounce; Mix them gradually, and when united, add Whale Oil, half a pint; and Stavesacre, in powder, half a pound: Mix all together into an ointment.

Figure 1.2.　An old recipe for treating lice in cattle.

Greeks persist today in Africa and India, where much of the farming is still at a nomadic or peasant stage of development. The intellectual members of the early communities took an intense interest in the details of disease, and from their descriptions can be recognized such diseases as foot and mouth and rinderpest. Foot-and-mouth disease too is still a major problem in South America, Africa and India and much of Europe, despite the development of modern control techniques involving the use of vaccines.

Controllable diseases are also still found throughout the world in the human field, with the continued clinical presence of tuberculosis, leprosy, malaria and the many forms of dysentery in the developing world. Human and veterinary medical knowledge have usually progressed in parallel, and many of the chemicals developed for use in the medical field have an application in animal therapy.

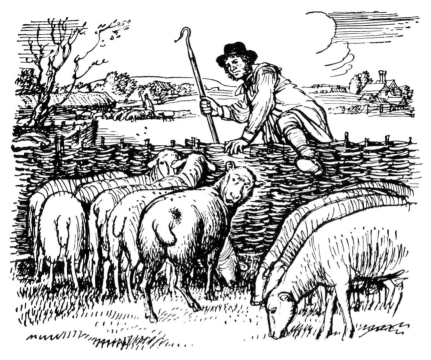

THE TREATMENT
OF FLY STRIKE

*Take Mercurial Sublimate, in powder, one ounce; Muriatic Acid, two ounces; Boiling
Water, three quarts; Put them all together in a stone bottle, and when cold, add Spirit of
Turpentine, one quart; One ounce of Tincture of Asafoetida: Mix and shake them well
together every time they are used.*

Figure 1.3.   An old recipe for treating fly strike.

Conversely, ideas formulated as a result of research in the control of
animal disease can frequently be applied in the human public health field,
because in many cases similar bacteria or viruses are involved. A major
advantage in disease control in animals, compared with much of human treatment, is that the animal patient will be given the medicine or the vaccine with
the ready consent of the farmer who is aware of the economic significance of
disease in his animals. The animal patient is also more likely to receive a
complete course of treatment as the drug has been paid for by the owner of
the animal.

Modern medicine

When Sir Alexander Fleming reported in 1929 on his finding that bacteria had been lysed by a fungus which had grown on an experimental plate, he produced the idea that started the scientific revolution in pharmacology and moved treatment in both the medical and veterinary fields from the empirical to the scientific. When it was later demonstrated that penicillin could be introduced into the body via the bloodstream with great safety, it gave confidence that other safe chemicals could be discovered for many disease conditions. In addition, with new techniques for blood assay, the course of a chemical within the blood and body tissues could be monitored from the moment of entry to its excretion via the kidney, gut or respiratory system. Before the discovery of penicillin, the majority of antibacterials, usually disinfectants, were too toxic to be applied other than to the outside of the body. The doctor and veterinary surgeon usually depended for their success both on the natural recovery powers of the body and on their ability to observe those signs and symptoms of disease which could indicate whether a favourable or unfavourable prognosis could be made.

In the immediate post-war period many of the drugs used for new human therapy were found to be suitable for application in animal treatment. Antibiotics and antibacterials, tranquillizers, anti-inflammatory drugs, anaesthetics and fertility control agents were all readily investigated for animal use. The arrival of the many new chemicals made possible the raising of the standards both of farming and of veterinary science, and provided the opportunity for the expansion of all aspects of animal production as it became possible to control or eliminate many of the diseases which had previously made animal production hazardous. The discovery of a range of new methods of chemical therapy thus made possible the gradual evolution of more effective animal farming.

Apart from the improvement in health of the animals, it became possible to improve their whole environment. In addition, a wider study began into the genetics of poultry, pigs and cattle, so that animals could be bred which were suitable for large-scale production.

Government control of new chemicals

As the use of new chemicals evolved, it became clear that controls must be established for their investigation and clinical testing before use. In the 1960s in the UK a committee on the safety of drugs (the Dunlop Committee) was established to act as a supervising, although voluntary, body for the control of all new drugs in the medical field. In parallel, a Veterinary Products Safety Precautions Scheme was devised to supervise the drugs which were to be sold directly to the farmer.

In 1968 a new law, the Medicines Act, was passed which established the principles that would be applied to the approval of all new and existing medicines which were to be used for the treatment and control of disease in man and animals. Similar legislation already had been evolved by the FDA in the United States, and members of the EEC in their different ways have gradually developed legislation which will provide a framework for the control of new drugs. This legislation is discussed in Chapter 11 in greater detail. The chemicals described in this book have all been accepted for animal use within the terms laid down by international drug legislation.

2. Animal disease in relation to the economics of animal production and to human health

The need for disease control

Until the discovery and subsequent development in the 1950s and 1960s of the range of completely new chemicals for use in animal treatment, the control of diseases on a national scale was considered important only if a disease posed an obvious recognized hazard to public health, or if the disease in animals was considered likely to decimate the animal population. Tuberculosis and rabies were obvious problems because of the danger they posed for human beings, and then it became urgent to control diseases which were known to be of great economic significance in the successful development of the animal industry, such as foot-and-mouth disease and brucellosis in cattle, swine fever in pigs and fowl pest in poultry.

Many other diseases of far greater economic importance to the individual farmer were tolerated by the authorities because they occurred on individual farms, and the responsibility for their control was considered to rest with the farmers. Into this category fell mastitis, a disease of the udder in dairy cattle, liver fluke and worm infestations in sheep and cattle and such diseases as *Salmonella* and *E.coli* infections in young pigs and calves.

At the same time it was recognized that the knowledge of the epidemiological and economic significance of these diseases was inadequate to justify strong policies of specific disease control.

Two major factors have radically altered our approach to disease problems in animals.

(1) The general acceptance of intensive systems for animal production highlighted the importance of diseases which had previously gone unrecognized or had been accepted as normal hazards in a small unit. Once records of disease incidence and economic returns were kept it soon became clear that disease outbreaks on large-scale farm operations could turn a previously successful farm into an uneconomic one. The search for cures or preventive systems for disease control became internationally important and veterinary research expanded both to determine the cause of disease and to develop control measures.

(2) The importance of diseases which can be transmitted from animal to

human has been recognized. As public health interest in possible hazards in food from animal sources increased, more and more zoonoses (infections which can spread to humans from domestic or wild animals) were recorded. Once a zoonotic disease was recognized (and there are well over 250) it became essential that its method of spread be defined, and ways and means of controlling it developed.

Intensive farming

The 1950s saw a major change in the management and farming of cattle, pigs and poultry—the new systems used have been variously called 'factory farming', 'intensive farming' and 'industrial farming'. These systems were developed initially in the USA to complement the large-scale grain farming which had been practised for many years in the wheat belts. The units were placed near the source of food so that transport costs were reduced to a minimum.

Poultry

It was recognized initially in poultry management that it was as easy to handle 10 000 animals as 50 or 100, if housing, feeding and breeding programmes could be planned on a bigger scale. To this end, housing systems were developed which allowed for the floor rearing of thousands of birds. Heat was supplied at strategic points throughout the house, and ventilation systems were introduced which ensured regular air changes.

This development was basically an extension of the brooding system for rearing chicks which had been practised first with paraffin heaters, then using gas or electricity to provide continuous heat over the first critical weeks when high temperatures are essential. It had been appreciated that the hen was not a very efficient rearer of her own chicks. Under natural conditions many of the chicks died in the first few days, either from extreme cold or as a result of bacterial or protozoal infections acquired from their mother during the first week of life. In addition, chicks born in the late autumn frequently could not withstand the severe winter conditions experienced in the American Mid West.

The experience gained from the intensive system for poultry also led to an appreciation of the importance of siting large animal-rearing systems close to the source of their food. The economic significance of this can be appreciated in the case of intensive cattle rearing, where the transport of large quantities of cattle feed can be expensive as 8 kg of feed are required for each 1 kg gain in weight. The success of large-scale poultry production undoubtedly provided the stimulus for the development of feed lots for cattle and larger units for pig production.

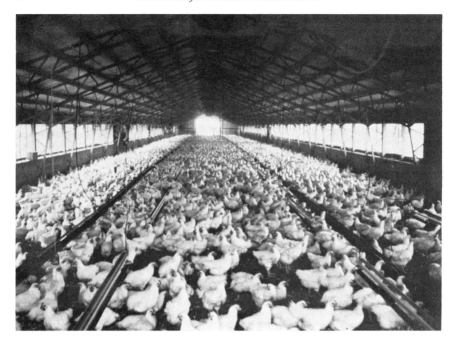

Figure 2.1.   Intensive rearing unit for poultry.

Cattle feed lots

Feed lots in Texas may feed and rear up to 50 000 cattle at a time. This has been possible only as a result of the use of modern methods of disease control and the careful recording of each animal during its time in a unit. Each animal on arrival at a feed lot is examined by a veterinarian and is vaccinated and treated for worm and other parasitic infections.

The feed lot cattle system depends on a continual supply of calves which may move into the feed lot at 6 months or 18 months of age. The total process from birth of cattle to slaughter can require one to two years. The breeding herds which produce the calves are usually located on pasture and range land, whereas the feed lot fattening units are usually found near cities where there is a dependable source of feed concentrates.

The cattle are kept in pens with an average of 400 square feet per animal – within the pen there is a common feeding and drinking facility. Fattening will take from 300 to 380 days.

Pig units

Pig units may now consist of 1000 breeding sows and these too have strict programmes of vaccination and parasite control.

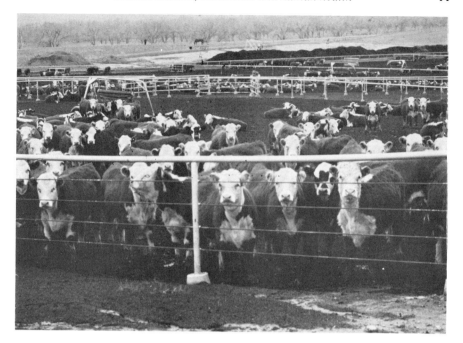

Figure 2.2.   A typical cattle feed lot in Texas.

The development of disease control

A feature of intensive systems is that special skills are needed in the farmer. He has to be a man who can recognize disease symptoms before an epidemic of disease has spread through a unit, and who has an appreciation of the importance of hygiene and preventive medicine in the control of disease. He also has to understand the economics of handling the housing, feeding and disease control of a large unit.

The previously largely practical activity of the rearing of animals has become a scientific operation which requires an understanding of a number of key subjects such as the epidemiology of disease, the importance of genetic selection of stock to develop the right type of animal for intensive management, and the specific nutritional requirements of rapidly growing stock.

The increase in broiler production in the USA that took place from 1950 to the 1970s, from 1×10^9 to 3×10^9 birds, was achieved as a result of basic changes in poultry production which were associated with (1) continued strain improvement, (2) improved disease control by the use of vaccines and coccidiostats and (3) improved housing and nutritional standards.

Similar patterns of development and improvement have occurred in the other intensive systems, such as in pig production, cattle feed lots and dairy units. The expansion in each area has been associated also with improved disease control techniques and new drugs.

Zoonoses as a human health hazard

Any disease of animals which can be a hazard as a result of regular contact between humans and animals ought to be eliminated. Where complete elimination of a disease is not possible, it is often practical to control bacterial or viral infections or parasitic infestations in animals by regular vaccination or drug treatment at strategic times.

Zoonoses are usually considered to belong to four different categories. These are:

(1) infections which pass directly from animal to human: *orthozoonoses*, such as brucellosis, salmonellosis;
(2) those infections in which an intermediate host such as an insect is involved, where there is a biological cycle in both the insect and the vertebrate host: *cyclozoonoses*, such as tick infestations;
(3) those in which infections result from accidental wound contamination: *metazoonoses*, such as anthrax;
(4) those which occur as a result of contamination of the soil or vegetation with viruses or bacteria: the *saprozoonoses*, such as *Salmonella*.

Zoonoses can, therefore, occur as a result of bacterial, viral or parasitic infections. In many cases the course of infection can be readily understood, but in others the source of infection is not so rapidly appreciated. For example, a rather unexpected zoonosis was found both in Australia and in New Zealand when *Salmonella* organisms were spread to sheep handlers in the 'outback'. Normally, salmonellosis is an oral infection spread when meat contaminated with organisms is eaten, but in Australia when large flocks of sheep were driven into collecting areas denuded of grass, the dust created was often contaminated with *Salmonella* organisms. Inhalation of this dust by the handlers then led to an acute respiratory infection due to the multiplication of *Salmonella* organisms in the respiratory system.

The more usual method of spread of *Salmonella* infection from animal sources to humans occurs when infected frozen poultry carcases or offal are prepared without thawing the frozen carcases thoroughly before cooking. If meat and poultry products are properly thawed out and adequately cooked, bacterial 'food poisoning' should not occur.

Public health and animal health

Over the last twenty years the maintenance of animal health has been recognized as important in its own right and also as a vital part of any public health disease control process. It is essential to maintain a healthy animal population within the intensive animal production systems if food is to be produced both safely and economically. In addition, it must be recognized that the presence of a wide range of zoonotic diseases within the animal population has placed a responsibility both on the public health and veterinary authorities to ensure that the epidemiology of each new disease is actively investigated. Once a disease is recognized, continued supervision must be maintained on any animal production area which could produce a health hazard.

Once it was appreciated that resistant strains of bacteria, helminths and insect parasites could occur and that they could cause cross-infection between animals and humans in the case of a zoonotic disease such as salmonellosis, control programmes for animals and humans had to be evolved. Fortunately, in the case of the gut bacterial infections of human beings, Hartley and Richmond (1975) have found that relatively few of the bacterial strains that flourish in the human intestines harbour resistance factors and that none of the strains that do can normally cause disease. When a patient or animal is taken off therapy with antibiotics, in the majority of infections the resistant strains are found to have disappeared from the gut. It has also been found that the effects of antibiotics on the bacterial flora vary from one individual to another.

Development of drugs for disease control

The development of drugs in the animal field, although initially influenced by the many new drugs which were specifically investigated for human use, soon evolved a pattern of its own. This was because disease control in animals must depend mainly on prevention rather than cure, whereas this was not always true in the human field. Disease on a farm, although often subclinical, could cause severe economic loss in a community.

Subclinical disease

Subclinical disease, or inapparent infection, can persist in two ways, as a *latent* infection or actively in a *carrier* animal. In either case, the potential for serious disease throughout an animal unit is alway present so that any programme of prevention must include the elimination of all forms of subclinical disease.

New drugs, therefore, had to be suitable for application to the whole herd or flock and required continual improvement or replacement to circumvent problems such as narrowness of spectrum of activity or resistance to a drug of the organism being treated. Because of this the number of drugs intended specifically for animal use has continued to increase over the last decade.

The changes that have taken place in animal production methods have opened up new fields of research which will both ensure the successful development of the new animal systems, and also clarify the relationship between human and animal disease. Intensive farming will be successful only if the new chemicals and vaccines are used to prevent rather than cure disease. It is in this respect that the problems of the modern animal unit often bear direct comparison with those posed in the human field in the prevention of disease and cross-infection in the surgical ward of a hospital, or in an army group in the field. The secret of success must lie in the prevention of the establishment of all communicable diseases within the animal or human community. This involves the use of chemical preventive therapy, such as anti-malarials in the human field and coccidiostats in poultry. The many different techniques will be discussed in Chapter 4.

3. The place of epidemiology in the planning of disease control programmes

Introduction

Epidemiology is the study of the factors associated with diseases in a human or animal population. The collective information on disease factors can provide the means of investigating and diagnosing disease in a community, and can then support the actions necessary to control disease.

The choice of methods used in establishing the pattern of disease in a particular animal unit or in a country will depend on a number of key factors:

(1) effective diagnosis of the disease;
(2) surveillance of outbreaks, including collecting data on disease incidence, establishing in which herds disease occurs, noting the effect of various methods of control on diseases and on disease incidence, studying the economics of disease control methods, etc.;
(3) establishing the relevance of the size of animal population to disease incidence and the number of staff required to oversee any outbreak.

Once an epidemiological study has been completed and a programme of disease control established, the success of any programme will depend on the implementation of a number of key control measures:

(1) A method of animal identification which is both comprehensive and accurate must be used.
(2) The farmer must maintain an effective recording system.
(3) A post mortem must be carried out on all dead animals and complete records kept.
(4) Quarantine must be applied to all new animal introductions to a farm.
(5) No change in management systems must take place without full discussion between the farmer and his veterinary surgeon.
(6) All major diseases such as brucellosis and tuberculosis must be already under control.

Effective control based on epidemiological studies

Smallpox

The application of epidemiological disease studies to diseases due to specific virus infections have demonstrated that the complete control and eradication of an important disease can be achieved. This is well illustrated by the successful elimination of smallpox as a notifiable disease of human beings. The first major step towards the containment of smallpox began when obligatory mass vaccination started seriously in Britain in 1940. Over the years international systematic vaccination and the enforcement of vaccination for all travellers rapidly reduced the incidence of smallpox. This was followed in most developed countries by a reliance on such epidemiological control systems as case detection, quarantine and selective vaccination of contacts for control in individual areas. The success of these initial measures made it possible to prepare a plan to achieve world control of the disease. The first step in this programme began when mass vaccination in endemic areas was recommended by WHO in 1967–68. A network of disease-reporting centres was established and programmes for the containment of specific outbreaks were initiated. In West Africa, it was found that surveillance and containment of disease pockets alone could eliminate disease even though smallpox incidence was still high. This finding allowed the primary emphasis in strategy to be shifted from mass vaccination to very specific control in certain areas.

Between 1967 and 1973 the number of countries in which the disease was considered to be endemic declined from 30 to 5. By 1973 it was possible to declare that the disease had been eradicated from the Americas and this was followed by elimination of smallpox from Africa and Eastern Asia by 1980.

In a similar fashion to smallpox, many animal diseases such as rinderpest and pleuro-pneumonia have been eliminated from endemic areas in Africa. Unfortunately, however, because of political instability, it is not always possible to maintain a state of complete freedom from disease, as control soon breaks down when one or other of the key aspects of the programme are not carried out (Rossiter *et al.* 1983).

Animal diseases

For our purposes, where we are referring to the use of drugs or vaccine therapy, animal diseases can be considered under a number of headings, dividing them into those diseases which must be controlled by a legislative process, and those which can be gradually overcome by the farmer's individual effort. All animal disease is economically important, but certain diseases pose special problems because of their high infectivity or their potential danger to the human handlers of the animals.

(1) *Epidemic diseases*: These are usually of international importance because, if they are left uncontrolled, in some countries sudden outbreaks of disease will occur in areas which have been free of the disease for many years. The majority of the diseases in this category are caused by viruses. Examples are foot-and-mouth disease, rinderpest, swine fever and rabies. These diseases can be controlled in individual countries by the types of measures described for smallpox: mass vaccination, surveillance and quarantine. Because animals are involved, selective slaughter programmes can speed up the process of eradication.

(2) *Serious endemic diseases*: These diseases usually occur in individual countries and their relative importance will depend on the controls applied locally. Examples are tuberculosis, brucellosis, Aujeszky's disease and leptospirosis.

(3) *Diseases of economic importance to the individual farmer*: Although of great economic importance to the individual farmer, certain diseases are not readily controlled by state schemes or vaccination programmes and depend for their control on the vigilance of each farmer. Examples are mastitis in dairy cattle, infectious bovine rhinitis and other respiratory infections in young cattle, foot rot in sheep, salmonellosis in all animals, swine dysentery in pigs, pig parvovirus, streptococcal meningitis in pigs, worm infestations in sheep and cattle, ectoparasite infestations in sheep and cattle, coccidiosis in poultry.

The diseases in class 3 are those which are most likely to be controlled by the use of chemicals and vaccines and, therefore, are often mentioned in this book. Some chemicals, such as disinfectants, may however be used in all three classes.

Control of disease

The prevention and control of a disease can be assisted in a number of ways once its epidemiological significance has been defined:

(1) By education of the population on the key aspects of animal diseases and their relationship to human problems.

(2) By the use of quarantine—that is, the isolation of diseased animals or the holding separately of imported animals to ensure that no occult disease exists. Quarantine in disease control has been practised very successfully by countries which are naturally isolated by the sea, or by a land frontier which can be controlled, for example, the USA, Canada, UK, Australia and New Zealand. Where quarantine controls are not applied, animal diseases can quickly spread from country to country, for example rabies by the movement of dogs, equine influenza by the movement of racehorses by air.

(3) By immunization, employing a vaccination policy against known diseases.

Table 3.1. The worldwide usage of chemicals and
biologicals in the animal health field.

Chemicals and biologicals	Usage % by dollar value
Anthelmintics	10
Antibacterials	12
Pesticides	6
Coccidiostats	5
Growth promoters	15
Nutritional supplements	25
Biologicals (vaccines and sera)	12
Miscellaneous pharmaceuticals	15

This is practised widely for the control of many bacterial and viral diseases
which affect animals.

(4) By good hygiene and disinfection programmes. The epidemiologist must
have established the cause of a disease and the means by which it is spread
if he is to recommend an effective disinfection programme. To this end
many countries have a register of disinfectants and a list of the infective
agents they will destroy.

(5) By chemotherapy, using the wide range of chemicals which have been
developed and investigated over the last thirty years. Table 3.1 lists the
major groups of chemical and biological agents which are now used for
animal disease control throughout the world and indicates their relative
usage based on the total values of each group sold. As a result of the
knowledge of disease control that has been acquired through epidemiological studies, chemicals and biologicals now play a key part in any programme for disease control.

The environmental complex

It is possible to evolve control programmes for the use of the chemical groups
described in Table 3.1 and Figures 3.1 – 3.5 illustrate how an environmental
complex diagram may prove useful in deciding what are the priorities to be
considered before a control programme is recommended.

The effective control of any disease will depend on the accumulated
knowledge gained from epidemiological studies. It is often useful to consider
diseases in the context of their environmental complex. This term is used to
emphasize that many factors in the environment interact both with the animal
species of central interest and with each other. These factors can be clearly
depicted in a diagram of overlapping areas (a Venn diagram), as in Figure 3.1
where the key elements of animal, disease agent and environmental factors
are shown—it is when the combination of detailed factors in each area occurs
that disease becomes established. Either expanding the circle with these
detailed factors, or drawing further overlapping circles for each, enables a

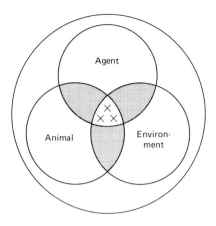

Figure 3.1.   Environmental complex diagram.
Shaded portions indicate areas of interaction. XX indicates area of disease.

clear picture to be built up of which factors may be important for the spread of disease in a particular environment.

The host (animal)

The host will carry all the genetic characteristics it has inherited from its parents. The initial immune response of the young animal will be inherited and consolidated after birth by the receipt of colostrum. It can be extended by vaccination against diseases known to occur within the environment.

Agents of infection

A range of infective organisms will exist within every system. Young animals can be protected from acute infection by being introduced into a farm unit under conditions most favourable to the host. Preventive treatment may be given during the introductory period. Good hygiene may eliminate or reduce the majority of infections before young animals are introduced into a farm unit.

A good example of how the life cycle of an important disease agent relates to factors in the host, and particularly in the external environment, is seen in the stomach worm of sheep (Figure 3.2). Infestations of several hundred mature worms can occur in adult sheep without producing any significant disease, but if the worm numbers rise to thousands or tens of thousands, illness and sometimes death can follow, particularly in lambs. The control of worm infestations must be primarily related to reducing the worm burden, and if it should be very heavy, to eliminating it by the use of an anthelmintic. Without treatment, the individual sheep, by passaging the worms through its

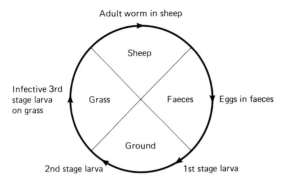

Figure 3.2.   Cycle of stomach worm infestation in sheep.

body, can increase the worm population very rapidly so that eventually the majority of the sheep in a flock may suffer stomach ulceration and anaemia due to loss of blood.

The adult female worms can lay up to 10 000 eggs per day for several months and the eggs are passed out in the faeces where they develop on the ground by moulting to the third larval stage (infective stage) within four days. The further rate of development of the larvae is then influenced by weather conditions. Warm moist conditions which favour growth of the grass and the development of the infective form will lead to the third stage climbing onto the grass which is then ingested by the sheep. A further larval moult takes place in the first stomach (the rumen) of the sheep and this fourth stage larva then migrates to the fourth stomach (abomasum) where it matures to the adult stage in about twenty days. The cycle is then restarted by the adult female laying eggs.

The significance of this life cycle to subsequent sheep infestations is dependent on many factors in the ecosystem. One is the state of the ground at the time an egg is passed out in the faeces. Many eggs may fail to hatch if the ground is parched and dry, and of those that do hatch, the rapidity of moult will depend on the warmth and moisture present on the ground and the grass.

Once the infective stage is reached, the rate of uptake of larvae by the sheep will depend on the number of sheep in a field and their grazing pattern. In addition, once the larvae reach the stomach and start to attach to the stomach wall, an immune response is stimulated within the sheep so that many larvae are rejected before reaching the adult stage.

From the life cycle pattern of a worm it is possible to estimate the numbers of worms and eggs in the sheep and the environment. These numbers are, however, much influenced by aspects of the ecosystem and the immune competence of the individual sheep. It is the epidemiologist's responsibility to take all these factors into consideration when he is formulating a worm control programme for a specific farm.

The environment

The influence of environment must be continually thought of in any intensive management system as it has a significant effect on the successful rearing of animals. For example, damp and cold houses can reduce growth response and may affect the ability of the young stock to resist disease. Bacteria and viruses frequently survive better in damp environments. The environment which surrounds animals must be controlled according to the number of animals in a house. In a broiler rearing house the atmosphere must be changed as the animals grow in size; for example, 10 000 day-old chicks require different conditions, in the same house, from those required by 10 000 eight-week-old chicks. Both will be present in the same house at the different stages of their development.

The range of factors in the environment which may need to be taken into account are shown in Figure 3.3 in the form of an expanded environmental complex diagram for the ecosystem of a dairy herd. The health and success of the herd can be affected by many factors such as the other animals on the farm, the state of the pastures, and the competition for space posed by such crops as cereals, roots and potatoes. Outside influences which are important are other farms and their disease patterns, the standard of hygiene maintained at markets at which cattle may be bought or sold, the cleanliness of delivery lorries and the effect of casual visitors such as hikers. In a well planned farm all these factors must be taken into consideration before new animals are brought on to the farm or expansion takes place.

The use of the environmental complex diagram

Three different disease problems have been chosen to illustrate how the environmental complex diagram can be helpful in highlighting the interdependence of host, agent and environment. Certain factors in each part of the complex have been identified as being of particular importance in the establishment of disease.

Mastitis in dairy cattle

This is a chronic and occasionally acute disease of the udder of the dairy cow which can, if neglected, cause serious economic loss to the farmer as a result of loss of milk and early culling of cows.

Host (dairy cow)

The majority of dairy cows are susceptible to the infective bacteria, although a small number are resistant. Susceptibility to infection can be influenced by

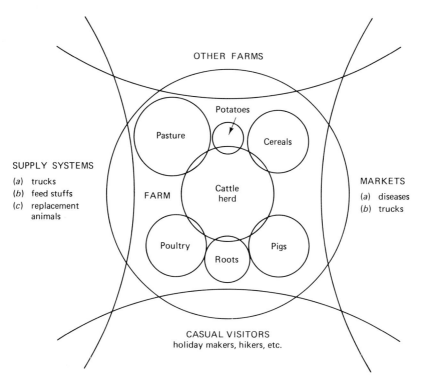

Figure 3.3.   Influences of ecosystem on a dairy herd.

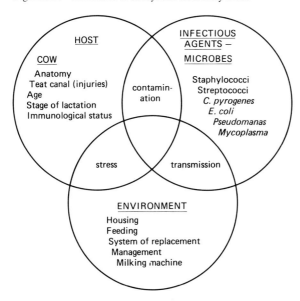

Figure 3.4.   Cow mastitis environmental complex.

genetic inheritance, by the age of the cow (most older cows carry persistent infections) and the anatomy of the udder and teats (pendulous teats can predispose to infection). All these factors have to be considered when maintaining the balance of population within a dairy herd.

Agents of infection

Many of the causal pathogens are ubiquitous but some are eliminated readily by antibiotic treatment. Others, such as staphylococci, can establish chronic infections in the udder and may produce strains which are resistant to certain antibiotics. The majority of the bacteria which invade the udder produce their most acute effect in a cow which is calving for the first time. *E. coli* organisms are particularly important at this time. Any control programme must aim at preventing infection entering the udder of the cow due to calve. In addition, all cows must have their calves in a clean environment.

Environment

One of the most important environmental influences is the milking machine, which must be cleaned and cleared of infection after each milking and must work at correct pressure. The housing must favour cow comfort and cleanliness and must be designed so that all cow standings can be cleaned easily every day.

Control

Based on a study of the factors in the environmental complex described for mastitis in a dairy herd, the National Institute of Dairying in Reading, England, evolved a control programme which is based on four key disease control practices. These are:

(1) maintenance of the milking machine;
(2) disinfection of the teats with an iodophor chemical solution following each milking to prevent new infections becoming established in the teat canal;
(3) treating all cows at drying off with an effective antibiotic formulation;
(4) treating all cases of mastitis with an antibiotic when they occur.

Calf enteritis

Host (calf)

Shortly after a calf is born it is exposed to the range of bacteria and viruses present in its environment, and its early response to these challenges will

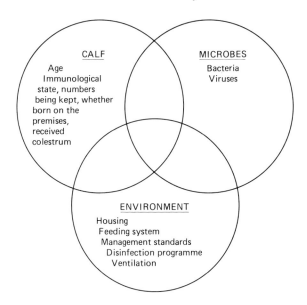

Figure 3.5.   Calf enteritis environmental complex.

depend on the antibodies it receives in the colostrum (first milk from its mother). In addition, if it is to be sold and moved to another farm during the first week of life, it will then be exposed to new pathogens and possibly active infections from other calves which are already on the new farm.

Agents of infection

Salmonella and *E. coli* are the major bacteria which may infect the young calf and two viruses, reoviruses and coronaviruses, may also play a part in the establishment of enteritis.

Environment

The housing must be designed specifically for handling young calves. This means that all concrete flooring must be readily drained, all walls and doors must be simple to disinfect and a microclimate must be established which is warm, but with adequate air movement to prevent excessive humidity.

The feeding regime must be a system which provides a balanced replacement for milk during the first period of growth, and the milk replacer must be of high quality.

Control

A control programme must include:

(1) provision of colostrum through early suckling of the cow followed by a nutritionally complete milk replacer when suckling is stopped;
(2) high standard of cleanliness, both in the immediate surrounds and in all utensils used for feeding;
(3) vaccination against *Salmonella* and *E. coli* where enteric infection has been recognized as likely within a unit;
(4) the use of appropriate antibiotic treatment should disease occur;
(5) should an enteric infection exist, fluid replacement by the use of a mixture of glucose, glycine and essential minerals should temporarily take the place of a milk replacer.

Pneumonia in weaned pigs

Host (pig)

Although disease occurs after the pigs have been weaned, the health of the sow is vital to the successful production of well developed weaned pigs, and great attention is now paid to her nutrition and housing and vaccination against known pathogens. The number of pigs kept by each sow must not exceed the sow's ability to feed them, and sows susceptible to 'farrowing fever' should not be kept in a herd.

Agents of infection

Pneumonia (enzootic pneumonia) is caused by a major causal agent *Mycoplasma hyopneumoniae*, and secondary bacterial invaders, *Pasteurella* species, *Haemophilus* species and *Bordetella*. Except where a unit is deliberately kept *Mycoplasma*-free, all these organisms are permanently present on many pig farms.

Environment

Control of the environment within a house will be a vital factor in control of pneumonia, with particular emphasis on batch size and controlled ventilation.

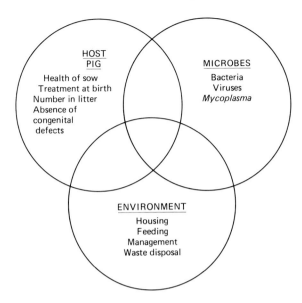

Figure 3.6.   Environmental complex for pneumonia in weaned pigs.

Control

Control of the disease must include the following elements:

(1) Establish *Mycoplasma*-free pig herds.
(2) Reduce the numbers of pigs kept in a house.
(3) Adopt an 'all in, all out' policy, i.e. each batch consists of weaners of the same age which are kept together throughout the rearing period. After the pigs leave the house it is disinfected and kept empty until the next batch arrives.
(4) Improve ventilation and air changes.
(5) Treat with antibiotics where a drug is likely to be effective. Where disease is regularly recognized, a 'growth promoter' may prevent the development of overt disease and will also assist in a good growth pattern.

4. Human and animal disease control and the method of use of chemicals

Introduction

In developed countries the major human infectious disease problems have been overcome by vaccination programmes, and by specific therapy for previously intractable diseases such as tuberculosis. The remaining problems now lie in areas such as cancer, mental illness, respiratory and circulatory problems (often associated with excessive smoking, overweight due to over-eating or lack of exercise), and accidents whether on the roads, at work or in the home.

This new position in the developed world is reflected in typical advertise-ments for pharmaceuticals which appear in the medical press. Five major areas of clinical problem predominate:

(1) malfunction of the central nervous system;
(2) hypertension—a problem of the circulatory system;
(3) arthritis and rheumatism;
(4) the gastric ulcer syndrome;
(5) bacterial diseases—mainly respiratory and intestinal infections.

As the majority of these clinical problems are associated with middle and old age it appears that the preventive medicine techniques associated with vaccination of the population and improvements both in nutrition and housing can deal with the major disease problems of youth.

In a paper on 'The Prospects for Prevention', Sir Richard Doll (1983) listed a number of areas which still provide scope for prevention of disease and early death in the UK:

(1) socio-economic improvements (housing, better nutrition etc.);
(2) modification of personal habits:
  (a) smoking
  (b) the abuse of alcohol and addictive drugs
  (c) improved diet
  (d) physical exercise;
(3) protection against accidents and their demands on the hospitals, for example, the use of seat belts in cars.

27

The fact that such areas were selected indicates the degree of sophistication that has occurred in human clinical medicine since the 1940s. This has largely been due both to advances in medical techniques and to the introduction of many new drugs. A modification of personal lifestyle is now almost more important than the cure of individual infections.

This pattern of disease prevention is in marked contrast to many of the requirements of medical knowledge in the developing nations, where survival in a hostile environment is still the main aim. The problems of the underdeveloped areas—the prevention of the existing diseases associated with malnutrition, poor hygiene and a variety of infections due to bacteria, viruses and external and internal parasites—bear a close resemblance to those associated with the raising of animals under both intensive and extensive systems. It is the fight against the many diseases caused by bacteria, viruses and external and internal parasites which is really important.

A list of the major pharmaceuticals advertised in the veterinary press reflects clearly the difference in emphasis between human and animal treatment. The major remedies advertised are usually for (1) antibacterials, (2) vaccines, (3) anthelmintics and (4) hormones for the control of the problems of reproduction. This would suggest that our animals are not yet neurotic, have little trouble with their heart and respiratory functions, do not suffer from gastric ulcers, but do have to be protected from ever-present bacterial, viral and helminth infections.

It is clear from the two patterns of disease described, that, with the exception of the developing countries, the major use of chemicals will differ between human and animal therapy and that the methods of application will in many cases be very different. In man, treatment is usually voluntary and can be given at set times to each individual patient and it is only in special circumstances, such as during a stay in hospital, that a drug has to be given by other than the oral route. Because of this, most new drugs in the medical field tend to be formulated as capsules or tablets for oral use or as fluids for injection; sometimes if a drug is unstable in the gastric juices it may always have to be given in an injectable form. It is then prepared for intravenous, intramuscular or subcutaneous use or as an intravenous drip.

In contrast, because of the variety of animal species which may have to be treated with a new chemical, the pharmacist who prepares a drug for animal use may have to formulate it in many different ways to satisfy the requirements both of the species of animal to be treated and the delivery system to be used. New methods of supplying drugs to animals may have to be designed to conform with the housing and handling methods practised with the animals.

Because the cat, dog and horse are expected to survive for their full life expectancy, treatment of these species tends to resemble that practised in the human clinical field. These animals are usually examined individually and, following diagnosis, are treated as individuals as they tend to be part of a human family. In the case of the other major species which require either therapeutic or preventive therapy, a wide variety of formulations and treatment systems have been developed to simplify handling while dosing. The important animal species on farms are (1) cattle—dairy and beef, (2) pigs of all ages, (3) poultry, both egg-layers and broilers and (4) sheep.

In most farm treatments, drugs are formulated in such a way that they can be given easily to large numbers of animals at a time, for example, in the water supply or in the feed. When given in this way they must be formulated so that an adequate dose of the drug will be provided to each animal and thus prevent the onset of specific disease. Such standard formulations for individual treatment of animals as tablets, powders, boluses and injectables have now been complemented by a wide range of specialized formulations and dosage systems which have been developed by teams of ingenious pharmacists, chemists, engineers and veterinarians. These new systems of dosing range from an oesophageal dosing gun for sheep which can place a drug directly in the rumen to metered water tanks which control the amount of a chemical to be added daily to the water supply of pigs and poultry.

Prolonged-release delivery systems

The prolonged release of drugs has a great attraction in animal therapy, in that it helps to overcome the problems of frequent mustering and handling of animals for treatment, and can provide a means by which a level of a drug can be maintained in the animals in a unit at key periods during a likely disease outbreak or when a metabolic imbalance problem has to be countered. The prolonged release can be achieved by a number of methods such as oral administration in the feed or water supply, external application to the skin, or by the injection or implantation under the skin of a slow-release formulation. One disadvantage of the continuous method of treatment is that once a regimen of treatment has been initiated, prompt termination of therapy is not possible should unexpected side-effects appear. It is essential also in the development of any prolonged release formulation to ensure that detectable levels of the drug do not persist either in the milk when sold or in the tissues when the animal is slaughtered for human consumption.

Oral prolonged-release formulations for ruminants

The concept of providing a long-acting drug for the ruminants (cattle and sheep) was first proposed and developed by Dewey, Lee and Marston (1958). They found that heavy foreign bodies when given orally were transported to the reticulum, one of the stomachs of the ruminant, and when dense enough remained there for several months. Their study involved the use of cobalt, an element which was not available in adequate quantities in the pasture in much

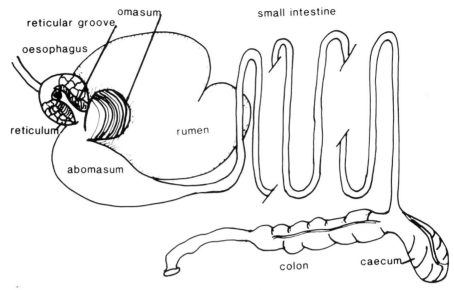

Figure 4.1.   Alimentary tract of ruminants – cattle and sheep.

of the sheep-grazing areas of South Australia, and the absence of which led to deficiency disease. Hard, dense pellets, or as they were more commonly known 'bullets', were prepared by baking cobalt oxide with china clay at a temperature of 1000 °C. From their resting place in the reticulum, the bullets released a steady supply of cobalt to be absorbed by the sheep over many months. This technique for supplying cobalt replaced the previous system of dosing sheep with a cobalt salt at least three times a week. The significance of this advance can be appreciated when it is realized that on some properties over 20 000 sheep might have to be collected and dosed at each treatment.

Other materials which have been used or can be used in this way are (*a*) copper, manganese and selenium, (*b*) anthelmintics, (*c*) antibloat agents, such as silicones, for cattle and sheep and (*d*) systemic insecticides. The original cobalt bullet system has in some cases been replaced by other ingenious devices for oral dosing which can remain in the rumen or reticulum and allow the slow release of specialized drugs.

Oral prolonged-release drug formulations for non-ruminants

Dichlorvos, an organophosphorus anthelmintic, has been prepared for slow release specifically in the horse and dog. When given orally in a simple dose form, it is highly toxic to the animals as it is absorbed too rapidly. When, however, it is incorporated in a resin in pellet form, it is so protected that it is slowly released as it passes through the stomach and intestine, and gives an anthelmintic effect without producing a toxic reaction.

Slow-release insecticidal formulations

A very practical slow-release insecticidal formulation can be provided in a dog collar. The insecticide is incorporated in thermoplastic resin and manufactured as a collar which is substituted for the normal collar daily during periods of insect exposure. This provides a slow-release medicament for the control of fleas, lice and ticks in dogs and cats. The insecticide is incorporated in one of two ways:

(1) A liquid insecticide with high vapour pressure is distributed throughout the collar, and the active principle slowly diffuses to the surface and is evaporated by the body warmth of the animal. An adequate concentration of the insecticide is present on and around the dog which is toxic to the pests but innocuous to the animal.

(2) A solid solution of the insecticide is present in the thermoplastic resin. The particles of the insecticide migrate from the formulation as a result of body movement and form a coating of particles of insecticide like a dust or powder on the surface of the collar. These then attach to the parasites and destroy them (Figure 4.2).

A similar thermoplastic resin formulation to that prepared for the dog collar has been incorporated in an ear tag for attachment to the inside of the ears of cattle in Africa. This destroys the ticks which attach to the ear in large numbers (Figure 4.3).

Prolonged-release formulations which act in specific parts of the body

A number of slow-release formulations have been developed which release active principles in various parts of the body:

(1) Vaginal sponge: this is an impregnated plastic sponge which contains the hormone methoxyprogesterone acetate. It is inserted into the vagina of ewes as a means of controlling the onset of oestrus. Removal of the sponge containing the hormone from treated ewes precipitates oestrus in a batch of ewes at one time. This allows batch lambing.

(2) Intra-uterine drug dispensers for antibacterial therapy.

(3) Slow-release formulations of antibiotics are prepared which are inserted into the udder of a cow via the teat sinus so that antibiotic can persist for two to three weeks in the milk channels during the dry period (non-milking stage of the udder). The antibiotic will eliminate the majority of the sensitive persistent bacteria which were present in tissues at the end of lactation.

(4) Teat sealants containing a bactericide are inserted into the teat canal during the dry period to prevent the entry of infections.

(5) Implants: a specialized formulation is implanted in the ear to allow the slow release of a hormone which will act as a growth promoter. This will be discussed in Chapter 9.

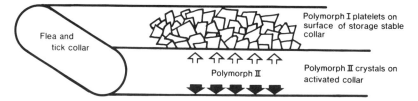

Figure 4.2.   Diagram of release of insectical crystals from a collar after activation on the neck of a dog. In this example, the platelet form of polymorph I crystals holds the pesticide inside the collar until disturbed, when the fine needles of the alternative polymorph II 'bloom' onto the surface and spread to kill the fleas and ticks.

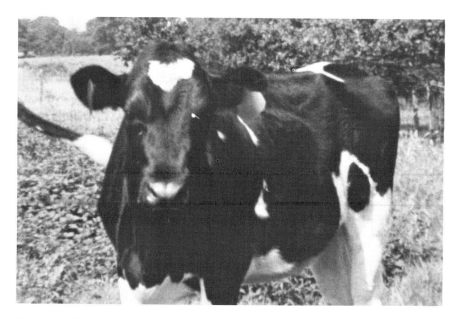

Figure 4.3.   Thermoplastic resin ear tag for control of ticks in ears of cattle.

'Pour-on' preparations

A novel 'pour-on' system for the application of a chemical is used for the control of warble fly infestation in cattle. The warble fly lays its eggs on the hair of cattle during August and September and the larvae which hatch then bore their way through the skin of the neck and head and move towards the area of the trachea and oesophagus where they continue to grow. They eventually move to the skin of the back where they create a hole and then fall to the ground to pupate, usually during March or April. This process leads to damage both to muscle tissue and to the hide, which reduces its value as a source of leather.

Organophosphorus insecticides, which are lethal to the larvae, when applied to the skin can penetrate to the tissues and reach a sufficient level in the serum to kill the larvae during the early phase (September/October) before tissue or skin damage occurs. When the insecticide in solution is poured evenly along the animal's back, it is absorbed and the migrating grubs are killed in all parts of the body.

Other chemicals such as anthelmintics are now being applied as 'pour-on' preparations to destroy helminth parasites in the intestines and other tissues of the body.

Oral pastes and liquid drenches

Both sheep and cattle, which graze either extensively or intensively, are exposed at some stages to oral infestation by worm larvae, which spend part of their life cycle on the blades or leaves of grass or clover. If infested animals are not treated with an anthelmintic and the infestations reduced, many will become anaemic and some will die; this can render uneconomic the keeping of sheep and, in some cases, cattle. To deal with this problem, veterinary research workers have concentrated on investigating ways and means of improving the activity of anthelmintics and simplifying their method of delivery. In parallel with these developments, studies of the life cycles of the various worms involved in disease have demonstrated that there are key times both of the year and of the age of sheep and cattle when treatment with an anthelmintic is likely to be most effective.

Initially, the method of treatment was to give each sheep a tablet or tablets, or dose it with a bottle containing anthelmintic. It was found, however, that some sheep which had appeared to swallow a tablet had merely placed it at the side of their mouth for it to be discarded later. Some hours after dosing, many tablets were found on the ground where they had been spat out by the sheep. Although a bottle was a satisfactory system for use with a few dozen sheep, it was quite impracticable when it came to dosing thousands on large farms in Australia or New Zealand. Specialized dosing guns were then developed which would automatically deliver repeatable doses. These guns were more effective still if attached by tube to a bag which carried twenty or more doses. Using this technique, several thousand sheep could be dosed each day as they passed through collecting pens.

The original simple solutions of carbon tetrachloride in oil, or suspensions of phenothiazine, were soon replaced with well formulated preparations of the newer anthelmintics which remain stable over a long dosing period. The experience gained in the preparation of emulsion paints has allowed development of paste formulations with the following characteristics:

(1) The paste is thixotropic (jelly-like until shaken or stirred, but then turning liquid).

(2) The paste is sufficiently sticky to ensure that it remains in the mouth at dosing.

(3) The paste is reasonably palatable.

(4) A high concentration of active principle is present in the paste so as to ensure that an adequate number of doses is present in each paste cartridge.

In addition to the paste formulations, many suspensions and liquids have been developed for delivery using a dosing gun—one example for intra-ruminal injection is shown in use in Figure 4.4.

Dips and spray races

In addition to carrying internal parasites, cattle and sheep are very susceptible to the attacks of a range of external parasites such as ticks, lice and blowflies. None of these parasites should be allowed to establish themselves on sheep or cattle; in sheep they will ruin the fleece and in cattle they will cause severe debilitation. Ticks, in addition to causing a considerable loss of blood, can transmit, while sucking blood, a range of protozoal organisms which can cause death or extreme debility.

It was soon recognized, particularly when cattle and sheep were introduced in large flocks in Australia, New Zealand, South Africa and South America, that regular control of parasites was necessary if disease losses were to be prevented. Until the discovery of effective pesticides, sheep and cattle were washed in running water and then in primitive dip baths containing arsenic or phenol emulsions.

The dip baths and tanks were gradually increased in size, and then in many countries spraying systems were introduced for the application of insecticides. As in the case of anthelmintics, insecticide formulations have been continually improved, so that they are now stable in dip baths and can be handled with safety.

Other systems of treatment

Other ingenious techniques have been developed for animal treatment and some of these are listed below.

(1) Aerosols—(a) insecticidal, (b) antiseptic, (c) intramammaries.

(2) Oral and inhalant vaccines.

(3) Teat sprays.

(4) Metering valves for providing measured doses of drugs.

(5) Copper needles which will remain in the abomasum of sheep and cattle for some months to counteract copper deficiency.

(6) Minerals such as copper, cobalt and selenium have been incorporated in soluble glass as a more effective bolus which may be given as a 'bullet' for retention in the rumen to release regular amounts of mineral.

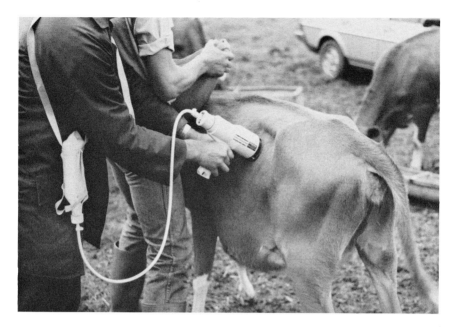

Figure 4.4.   Intraruminal injection of anthelmintic.

Conclusion

The developments described have been evolved over the years as a response to necessity and, in the case of sprays, the experience gained in the application of spray materials to both crops and fruit trees has been invaluable. It is gratifying to see the way in which research workers from a variety of disciplines can work together to produce equipment which is evolved step by step in association with chemical research.

5. Antibacterials and antibiotics

Introduction

It is difficult to appreciate that it is only about 40 years since the introduction for general usage, both for human and animal treatment, of the early antibacterials and antibiotics which revolutionized the therapy of bacterial infections. Chemotherapy played only a small part in clinical medicine until the introduction of Prontosil, the forerunner of the sulphonamides, in 1935. The sulphonamides were followed within five years by penicillins and later by many other antibiotics, each extending the scope of antibacterial treatment to infections which until then were insusceptible. At the same time other synthetic compounds were introduced, including more sulphonamides, important anti-tuberculosis drugs, and others with a limited utility in infections of the urinary and alimentary tracts. These innovations have changed the pattern of infectious disease in two ways. They have greatly reduced the severity and the mortality from infections and, in some cases, the incidence of many bacterial diseases.

As with human treatments, dramatic results have been achieved in the last 40 years in the field of therapy of animal disease. Diseases such as bacterial mastitis in the dairy cow, bacterial enteritis and pneumonia in animals of all ages have now become manageable. Foot and leg infections in cattle, sheep and horses due to bacteria, in the past often caused continual ill health and, in many cases, death. Without the antibacterials and antibiotics it would not have been possible nor could it have been justified economically to build up the animal production industry to the present position where it provides food for the whole population. Before the war of 1939–45 animal production in the UK, for instance, was a relatively small industry and most of the food for Britain came from New Zealand, Australia, Argentina, the USA, Denmark and Holland. The improved farming methods that became necessary during the war and the rapid expansion of the dairy herd which followed were dependent to a large extent on advances in the methods of disease control.

The chemicals which will be discussed in this chapter can, therefore, be considered as important tools which played a vital part in the successful development of animal production throughout the world. The importance of these drugs and their effect on the health of farm animals can readily be appreciated when it is realized that the modern healthy dairy cow produces twice as much milk as its pre-1940 counterpart, and the modern roasting chicken is produced in 7–8 weeks whereas its predecessor would have taken at least 14 weeks to be ready for the table. Beef can be produced in 10–12 months compared with 3 years pre-war. These developments occurred quite rapidly, so that effective disease control had to run in parallel with the improvements in animal breeding and nutrition.

As was discussed in Chapter 3, many of the major diseases in animals which still have to be controlled are due to bacterial infections. It is important, therefore, that the effective techniques for the use of antibacterials must be understood, and they must not be used carelessly so that patterns of resistance develop which might vitiate the value of a very effective chemical. In this chapter the general principles of antibacterial therapy are discussed first, then the individual chemicals which are now available.

Source of antibiotics and antibacterials

As a result of the discovery and successful development of penicillin, it was decided by many international pharmaceutical companies, and also government-funded research centres, that it would be rewarding to carry out soil surveys in the hope of finding new antibiotics with wider properties or specific activity which were not present in penicillin. Most antibiotics are metabolites of bacteria or fungi and have been discovered either as a result of chance observation or following the screening of large numbers of soil samples.

In addition, synthetic antibiotics have often been discovered by examining compounds related to existing active materials for new or improved activity. Much has been achieved in this way, and it has frequently been assumed that the ultimate in activity has been reached, but there are still areas of disease which require more effective drug activity. Some of these are:
(1) greater activity against *Pseudomonas* and a wider spectrum in all drugs including activity against resistant bacteria;
(2) better persistence in the tissues and the penetration of chemicals to difficult sites such as joints and the central nervous system;
(3) activity against combined bacterial and viral infections.

Assay of antibacterials

Antibacterials are assayed either biologically or physicochemically.

Biological assay is carried out by the use of an agar-based medium which has been seeded with a specific strain of organism sensitive to antibiotic activity at a low level.

Physicochemical techniques for the detection of antibacterials now include spectrophotometry, spectrofluorimetry and high-performance liquid chromatography. These methods are not always as sensitive as biological assays, but are preferred by the drug registration authorities as they are considered to be less dependent on individual human interpretation.

Sensitivity tests for in vitro studies

Sensitivity tests of individual bacterial species are often carried out before animal treatment is initiated, using sensitivity discs which are available for the majority of antibiotics in common use. Paper discs containing known quantities of antibiotic are placed on a Petri dish containing agar-based medium onto the whole surface of which the organism under test has been inoculated (Figure 5.1). The bacterial culture must be a pure one of the organism to be tested. One disadvantage of the disc test is that 24–36 hours may pass before a result is known, as the bacteria have to be isolated in pure culture before the plate is seeded.

Minimum inhibitory concentration

The minimum inhibitory concentration (MIC) of an antibiotic required to inhibit the growth of a bacterium is established by growing the organism in a range of dilutions of the antibiotic. The lowest concentration which prevents visible growth of bacteria is taken as the MIC. That level is then related to the dose of drug which will be used in the treatment of clinical infections.

Mode of action of antibacterials

As antibacterials have been discovered and developed, knowledge of their mode of action has been accumulated. It is now considered that they can influence various aspects of the synthesis and development of parts of the bacterial cell, of which the principal ones are:
(1) the nucleic acid content;
(2) protein synthesis of the cell;
(3) the formation of the cell wall;
(4) cell membrane development.

Influence on nucleic acid content

Replication of the nucleic acids of the bacterial cell is prevented directly by some antibacterials and indirectly by the sulphonamides.

Protein synthesis of the cell

Streptomycin, tetracyclines, the macrolides and lincomycin all act by interfering with the normal development of the protein combinations necessary for bacterial growth. In the growth phase, the process of linking together amino acids to form a new bacterial cell has to proceed in a cyclical fashion.

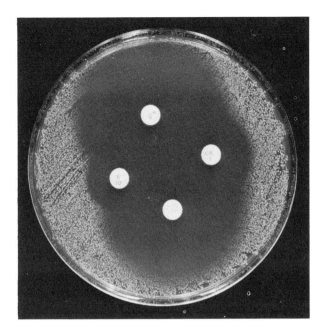

Figure 5.1. Assays for antibiotic action. An agar plate uniformly seeded with the bacteria is incubated with a disc containing the antibiotic which diffuses out from the disc, leading tom a concentration gradient. Antibiotic-sensitive bacteria are inhibited by quite low concentrations so can only grow if far from the antibiotic disc; resistant ones can withstand much higher amounts of antibiotic, so are found much closer to the disc.
A zone of inhibition does not necessarily imply significant sensitivity, unless the area is as large as that of a known sensitive strain of the same organism.
(a) *Staphylococci* sensitive to the four antibiotics penicillin G (P), streptomycin (S), ampicillin (AM) and chloramphenicol (CX) have grown only around the edge of the plate.
Further examples are shown in Figure 5.1(b)–(e) on the following pages.

Any interruption of the cycle locks the process at the point of interference and growth is halted.

The formation of the cell wall

The cell wall of a bacterium is rigid and lies outside the cell membrane, giving the cell protection from possible osmotic damage. Such a cell wall is absent from mammalian cells, so that an agent which influences the cell wall formation in bacteria will not necessarily have a damaging effect on the mammalian host. Both penicillins and cephalosporins affect cell wall synthesis.

Most antibiotics which act on cell walls interfere with the later stages of the cell wall synthesis. Thus, penicillin and cephalosporin inhibit the final cross-linking of the glycine and peptide chains. When penicillin is present, the cell membrane of the new bacterium is progressively deprived of external support as the wall which is being built weakens. The cell ruptures because it can no longer withstand the osmotic pressure inside it.

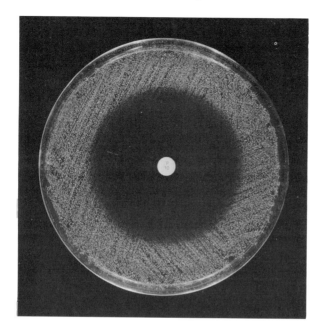

(b) The sensitive *Staphylococci* have been inhibited by penicillin as far as two thirds of the plate's radius, whereas in (c) the resistant *Staphylococci* can grow almost up to the penicillin disc.

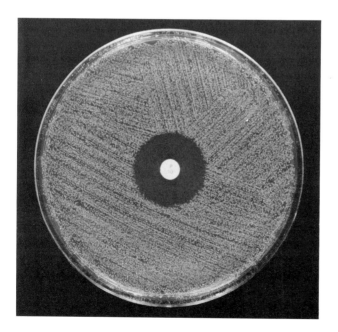

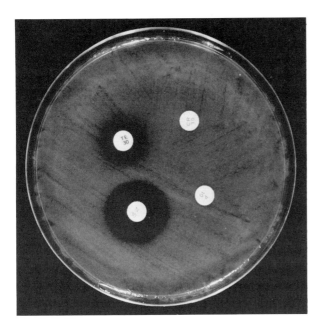

(*d*) A *Pseudomonas* strain resistant to penicillin G (P) and chloramphenicol (CR) is not affected by these drugs but is inhibited by tetracycline (TE) and neomycin (N).

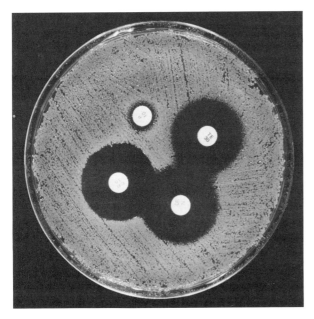

(*e*) A strain of *Escherichia coli* resistant to penicillin G (P) but sensitive to tetracycline (TE), neomycin (N) and chloramphenicol (CR).

Cell membrane development

Beneath the cell wall is a lipoprotein layer of cell membrane. The peptide antibiotics act by attaching to the membrane and modifying the flux of magnesium ions through it, which brings about lysis of the cell.

Methods of describing antibiotics and antibacterials

Antibiotics and antibacterials are described in various ways according to their structure, their mode of action and their range of activity.

(1) They may be classified by chemical structure, such as β-lactam antibiotics (penicillins, cephalosporins); aminoglycosides (neomycin); tetracyclines (chlortetracycline); sulphonamides (sulphanilamide); macrolides (tylosin).
(2) They may also be described as bacteriostatic if they only halt bacterial growth (stasis) or bactericidal if they actually kill the bacteria.
(3) For other purposes they are described as having narrow or broad-spectrum activity, according to the range of bacteria which each individual antibacterial will attack. This will be mentioned later as individual antibiotics are discussed.
(4) They may be described as being effective mainly against either Gram positive or Gram negative bacteria, a classification which depends upon the organism's response when fixed and exposed to the dye formulation evolved by Hans Gram, a Danish physician. This is a differential staining method using the retention or lack of retention of a purple dye. Gram negative organisms show as red under the microscope and Gram positive as blue.

Clinical use of antibacterials

Several important aspects of the behaviour of an antibacterial agent within the body have to be assessed before a suitable formulation can be evolved for clinical use.
(1) The blood and tissue levels of available antibiotic have to be adequate at all sites of likely bacterial infection.
(2) The antibiotic should not be reduced in activity in the presence of serum, blood and pus.
(3) The antibiotic should be able to cross the main physiological barriers in adequate concentrations to be effective, for example, blood–brain, placenta, intestinal barrier, mammary tissue for action in milk.

Tables 5.1–5.5 list some of the major infections found in animals in which bacteria play a part. The value of existing and new antibacterials is related to their activity against these organisms, and the economic part an antibacterial plays in the treatment of an animal.

Table 5.1.   Major bacterial infections of cattle.

Disease	Major bacteria involved	Gram + or Gram −
Calf enteritis and pneumonia	*E. coli*	−
	Staphylococci	+
	Pasteurella	−
	Salmonella	−
Mastitis	*Staphylococci*	+
	Streptococci	+
	E. coli	−
	Pseudomonas	−
	Corynebacteria	+
Metritis	*E. coli*	−
	Staphylococci	+
	Streptococcus faecalis	+
	Proteus	−
Pyelonephritis	*Corynebacterium renale*	+
Bovine infectious keratitis	*Moraxella bovis*	−
Foul in the foot	*Fusiformis* spp.	−
Wooden tongue	*Actinobacillus* spp.	−

Table 5.2.   Major bacterial infections of pigs.

Disease	Major bacteria involved	Gram + or Gram −
Enteritis and pneumonia	*E. coli*	−
	Salmonella	−
	Pasteurella	−
	Haemophilus	−
	Bordetella	−
	(*M.hyopneumoniae*) (mycoplasma)	
Erysipelas	*Erysipelothrix rhusiopathiae*	+
Metritis	*E. coli*	−
	Staphylococci	+
Meningitis	*Streptococcus suis*	+

Table 5.3.   Major bacterial infections of horses.

Disease	Major bacteria involved	Gram + or Gram −
Enteritis and septicaemia in the young foal	*E. coli*	−
	Proteus	−
	Staphylococci	+
Strangles	*Streptococcus equi*	+
Metritis	*E. coli*	−
	Staphylococci	+
Contagious endometritis	*Haemophilus equigenitalis*	−
	E. coli	−
	Klebsiella	−
	Pseudomonas	−
Pneumonia	*Staphylococci*	+
	Pasteurella	−

Table 5.4.   Major bacterial infections of poultry.

Disease	Major bacteria involved	Gram + or Gram −
Coli septicaemia	*E. coli*	−
Salmonellosis	*Salmonella* spp.	−
Mycoplasmosis	*Mycoplasma*	
Staphylococcosis	*Staphylococci*	+

Table 5.5.   Major bacterial infections of dogs and cats.

Disease	Major bacteria involved	Gram + or Gram −
Enteritis	*E. coli*	−
	Salmonella	−
Ear infections	*Staphylococci*	+
	Streptococci	+
	E. coli	−
	Pseudomonas	−
Skin infections	*Staphylococci*	+
Leptospirosis	*Leptospira canicola*	
Respiratory infections	*Staphylococci*	+
	Streptococci	+

Bacterial resistance

One of the inevitable results of using an effective antibiotic is that it will kill or render static most of the sensitive organisms it comes in contact with, but the majority of the resistant strains will be unaffected. These will have to be disposed of by the body's normal immune mechanisms. Frequent use of an antibiotic in a specific environment can lead to a temporary dominance of resistant bacterial strains. The likelihood of this occurring depends on the antibiotic used, the natural incidence of resistant strains within the environment and for how long the antibiotic therapy is applied.

Resistance can develop during therapy or naturally for a number of reasons:

(1) mutation—this can occur spontaneously in nature whether or not therapy is being applied;
(2) acquisition of resistance genes (infectious drug resistance)—this can occur where contact occurs between two bacteria and the gene for resistance of one is passed to the other;
(3) cross-infection—this occurs as a result of the acquisition by the animal under treatment of new organisms which may be resistant;
(4) selection of resistant variants from within the animal under treatment.

It is important, therefore, when large numbers of animals are being treated to be aware of the possibility of resistance developing during treatment as a result of therapy. The veterinary clinician has a responsibility to monitor the bacterial pattern on a farm, and to ensure that he uses effective antibiotics and does not persist with a specific antibiotic when resistant strains to it are well established.

Sulphonamides

Prontosil, the first of the chemical structures containing the *p*-aminosulphonamide group, was shown to have antibacterial activity in 1935. It was also found that Prontosil was metabolized in the body and excreted in the urine in the form of sulphanilamide, so that it seemed likely that sulphanilamide was the antibacterially active portion of Prontosil. Further work using mice which had received a lethal dose of bacteria showed that sulphanilamide was indeed a potent antibacterial chemical.

This discovery stimulated a research programme which led to the synthesis of several thousand derivatives of sulphanilamide. The nucleus of the sulphonamides has a close resemblance to *p*-aminobenzoic acid, an essential member of the vitamin B complex. The sulphonamides act against bacteria by substituting and displacing the essential vitamins which are necessary for the survival of the bacteria.

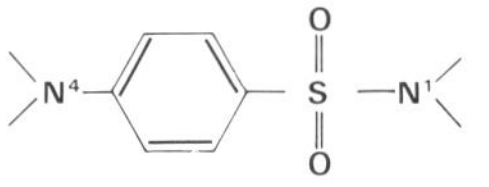

Sulphonamide nucleus

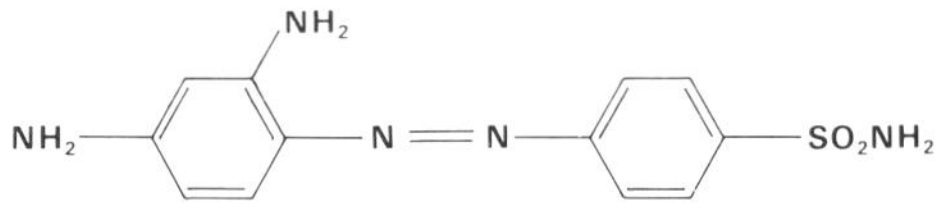

Prontosil®

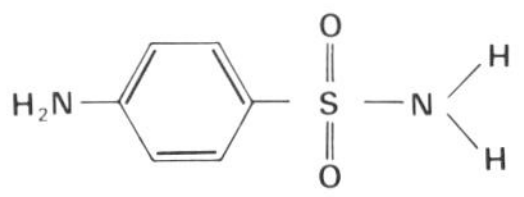

Sulphanilamide (*p*-aminobenzene sulphonamide)

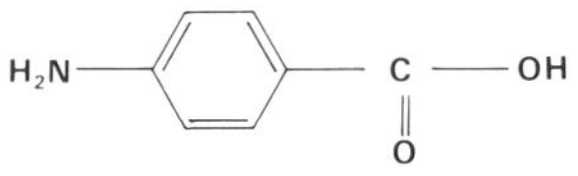

p-Aminobenzoic acid

The sulphonamides that have been prepared for use in veterinary therapy can be considered in two main groups:
(1) systemic sulphonamides, which are absorbed from the intestines and so can act throughout the body, and
(2) gut-active sulphonamides, which are poorly absorbed from the intestines and exert their effect mainly on the intestinal flora within the gut.

Systemic sulphonamides

The therapeutic activity of the sulphonamides is dependent on their solubility in water, as the concentrations they will achieve in the tissues are related to their rates of absorption.

The systemic sulphonamides most commonly used in animals are: sulphanilamide, sulphacetamide, sulphapyridine, sulphamethazine, sulphathiazole and sulphaquinoxaline.

The pharmacological actions of the sulphonamides tend to be very similar. Once absorbed, they are rapidly distributed throughout the bloodstream to the various tissues and fluids by passive diffusion. A dynamic equilibrium is established between the sulphonamide in the blood and both the extracellular and intracellular fluids. The equilibrium is most rapidly established in tissues which are highly vascular.

Sulphonamides can cross the blood–brain barrier, and also diffuse into the milk when given orally or intravenously.

Metabolism

Sulphonamides are metabolized in the body mainly by acetylation and conjugation, and are then excreted in the urine, faeces and milk.

Their activity in the body is determined by blood concentration—a level of 5 mg per 100 ml of blood is recognized as therapeutically effective. It is usual when treating a patient to rapidly establish a therapeutic blood and tissue level by giving an initial large dose and this is followed by smaller doses. The initial large dose is necessary because the availability of sulphonamides is variable as a result of protein binding and acetylation in the liver.

Antibacterial action

The sulphonamides are active mainly against Gram-positive organisms such as staphylococci and streptococci, but some sulphonamides have good activity against Gram-negative organisms such as *E. coli*.

Animal treatment

The systemic sulphonamides are still widely used in animal treatment for such conditions as bacterial pneumonia, septicaemia and enteritis, particularly in young animals such as calves. Sulphamethazine is particularly useful in the treatment of 'foul in the foot', a disease of adult cattle.

Gut-active sulphonamides

The members of this group have been selected for oral use because they have low water solubility and are poorly absorbed from the gut. They include succinylsulphathiazole, phthalylsulphathiazole and sulphaguanidine.

The first two are hydrolysed in the intestines to release respectively (*a*) succinic acid plus sulphathiazole and (*b*) phthalic acid plus sulphathiazole. The sulphathiazole then acts on the intestinal bacteria.

Sulphaguanidine is poorly absorbed because it is ionized at the pH of the gut. Many of these drugs have now been replaced in animal therapy by the more active antibiotics.

Potentiated sulphonamides

Following wide usage of sulphonamides, strains of resistant bacteria became common, and it was found that resistance to one sulphonamide meant resistance to the others in the group. It was important, therefore, if the sulphonamides were to remain in use, that a means of protecting the sulphonamides or enhancing their activity must be found.

In the 1960s it was reported by Hitchings (1961) that it was possible to widen the action of the sulphonamides by combining them with inhibitors of bacterial dihydrofolate reductases. A particularly useful inhibitor was found to be trimethoprim which had been used as an antimalarial in combination with a sulphonamide. When trimethoprim is administered at the same time as a sulphonamide, together they inhibit the formation and reduction of bacterial dihydrofolic acid—an essential development for bacterial survival. The blockade produced by the combination of the two chemicals leads to an antibacterial action which is greater than the separate effect of the individual compounds. Table 5.6 shows the effect of the combination of trimethoprim and sulphadiazine on a number of animal pathogens which would otherwise have been resistant.

It has been found after wide usage that resistance can develop even to this combination, so that it is important to determine the sensitivity pattern of the chemicals on a farm before using the combination.

Table 5.6. Minimum inhibitory concentrations of trimethoprim, sulphadiazine and combinations against various bacteria.

Organism	Alone		In combination	
	Trimethoprim MIC	Sulphadiazine MIC	Trimethoprim 1 part MIC	Sulphadiazine 5 parts MIC
E. coli	0·63	>250*	0·31	0·4
	10	>200*	0·31	6·25
Staph. pyogenes	5	>200*	1·25	1·56
	5	>200*	0·16	6·25
Strep. agalactiae	5	>200*	0·04	25
	12·5	>250*	0·2	2
Strep. dysgalactiae	3·12	25	0·31	3·12
	3·12	>250*	0·4	125
Strep. uberis	0·31	0·2	0·0025	0·2
	1·25	3·12	0·0025	1·56

*Indicates organisms are resistant to sulphadiazine if the drug is given on its own.

The penicillins and cephalosporins (β-lactam antibiotics)

The term β-lactam antibiotics is now applied to penicillin and the many new penicillins which have been developed since Fleming's original report in 1929 on the activity of penicillin against pathogenic staphylococci. It is also applied to the range of cephalosporins which were first described by Newton and Abraham (1956).

The basic structure of the penicillins and cephalosporins centres on the four-membered β-lactam ring. In penicillin, the β-lactam ring is fused to a five-membered thiazolidine ring. The thiazolidine ring is comparatively stable, but the β-lactam ring is very unstable and can be readily broken chemically (for example, by gastric hydrochloric acid) or enzymically by penicillinases (β-lactamases) produced by certain penicillin-resistant bacteria. The nature of the side-chain R can affect the penicillinase-resistance of the molecule as well as many of its other biological and chemical properties.

β-lactam ring

five-membered thiazolidine ring

Penicillin structure

β-lactam
ring

six-membered
thiazine ring

Cephalosporin structure

In the case of the cephalosporins, the β-lactam ring is fused to a six-membered ring. These new antibiotics had an initial advantage in that the β-lactam ring was resistant to hydrolysis by certain β-lactamases produced by bacteria.

Since the first report by Fleming of antibiotic activity from *Penicillium* mould and the subsequent work by Florey and Chain which led to the isolation of penicillin, a whole range of penicillins have been developed. Several naturally occurring variants were found, but a much greater broadening of penicillin's activity was made possible by the isolation of 6-aminopenicillanic acid by Batchelor *et al.* (1959). An almost unlimited variety of side-chains R could be linked chemically to the free amino (NH_2) group.

Figure 5.2 gives a diagrammatic picture of the discovery of the many new active penicillins which followed the separation of the nucleus. New cephalosporins also have appeared in regular succession, as it has been possible to add side-chains to the nucleus.

Despite the chemical research which led to the development of the range of new penicillins and cephalosporins, it is still most economical to obtain the nucleus of both penicillins and cephalosporins by fermentation from fungal growth of *Penicillium* and *Cephalosporium* in large vats.

Mode of action

Penicillins act specifically by interfering with the development of the bacterial cell wall. The enzyme transpeptidase is rendered inactive, so that it cannot form the cross-linkage necessary between two linear peptidoglycan strands, the main structural components of the cell wall.

Because they act so specifically on cell wall development the penicillins affect only growing cells. They therefore show their greatest activity when bacterial multiplication is highest and have little action when the bacteria are dormant. In addition, penicillins have no adverse effect on mammalian tissue because the mammalian cells do not possess a rigid wall structure.

Spectrum of activity

The original penicillin G had a number of therapeutic weaknesses.
(1) It had poor activity against Gram negative bacteria.

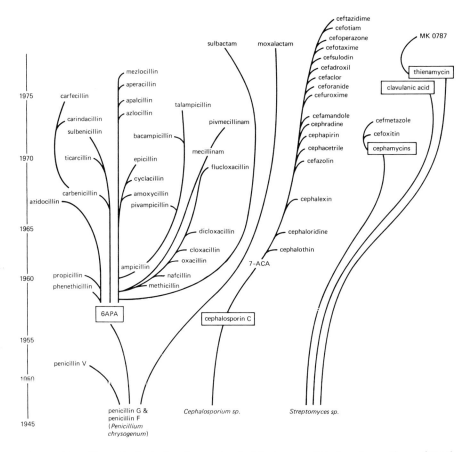

Figure 5.2. Chronological development of β-lactam antibiotics from three fungal species—*Penicillium, Cephalosporium* and *Streptomyces*. Based on a scheme by G. Rolinson.

(2) It was destroyed by the acid of the stomach.

(3) It was destroyed by the β-lactamase enzyme penicillinase which is produced by many strains of the target bacteria.

Table 5.7 indicates how penicillins differ in activity and why it was necessary to develop the wide range of penicillins now in use in both the medical and veterinary fields. Column (1) represents the original penicillin G which is destroyed in the gastric juices and has to be given by injection; it is also very sensitive to penicillinases. Column (2) represents the very specific penicillins which are resistant to penicillinases but still have a narrow spectrum. Column (3) represents a genuinely broad-spectrum penicillin and Column (4) represents a specific antipseudomonas penicillin.

Table 5.7. Minimum inhibitory concentrations of penicillins against various bacteria.

| Organism | Minimum inhibitory concentration (μg/ml) | | | |
	(1) Penicillin G narrow spectrum	(2) Cloxacillin penicillinase stable	(3) Ampicillin broad spectrum	(4) Carbenicillin anti- pseudomonas
Staphylococci 'S'	0·02	0·1	0·05	1·25
Staphylococci 'R'	R	0·25	R	25
Streptococci	0·01	0·1	0·02	0·5
Clostridium welchi	0·05	0·5	0·05	0·5
Haemophilus influenzae	0·5	12·5	0·25	0·25
E. coli	50	R	5	5
Salmonella	2·5–16	R	1·25	2–16
Proteus	5	R	1·25	2·5
Klebsiella	250	R	250	250
Pseudomonas	R	R	R	50

R (resistant) = an MIC greater than 250 μg/l.

The range of penicillins particularly suitable for use in animal treatment include penicillin G, amoxycillin, ampicillin, carbenicillin, cloxacillin, nafcillin and pivampicillin.

Pharmacokinetics

As the mechanisms of antibacterial activity of all penicillins are similar, the major differences lie in variations in absorption and excretion patterns.

Penicillins are usually prepared as the sodium salt and are rapidly absorbed from the site of a parenteral injection. Effective blood levels are reached within 30 minutes of injection and the antibiotic is then distributed throughout the body. The level of antibiotic reached throughout the body will vary according to the dose given, and penetration of certain barriers, in particular the blood–brain barrier and the placenta, may require higher blood levels. Some newer penicillins are much more acid-resistant than the natural ones and are well absorbed from the gut, so that oral dosing is effective except where exceptionally high levels of antibiotic are required.

All the penicillins are excreted readily through the kidneys, so that penicillins are particularly useful for urinary infections where high levels of antibiotic are necessary. Certain slow-release preparations of penicillins have been prepared by using relatively insoluble salts mixed with slow-release substances such as aluminium monostearate. These are useful where a prolonged effect is required, such as in mastitis treatment or other chronic infections.

Toxicology

Because of penicillin's lack of action on mammalian tissues, toxic reactions following its use in animal therapy are uncommon.

Clinical use

Cloxacillin

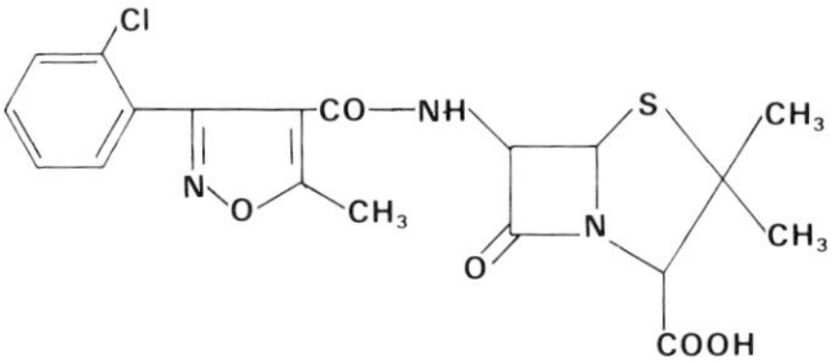

Cloxacillin was one of the first of the new penicillins to be used for animal therapy, as it is stable to staphylococcal penicillinase and is active against the range of Gram-positive organisms, including *Staphylococcus aureus*, which cause mastitis in dairy cattle. Its major use is for the treatment of mastitis and particularly in a slow-release form for the treatment and prevention of mastitis during the dry period. For the latter purpose, cloxacillin is prepared as the relatively insoluble benzathine salt in an oil base and is inserted via the teat canal into the udder at the end of lactation when cows are 'dried off'. Drying off is the cessation of milking, which is practised for an eight-week period during the latter stage of pregnancy. Milk production restarts at calving.

Ampicillin and amoxycillin

These two penicillins can be considered together as they have similar anti-bacterial activity, but amoxycillin is better absorbed when given by mouth. It also has a more rapid and complete bactericidal effect, because it interferes very rapidly with cell wall formation and causes the formation of spheroblasts and lysis of the cell.

This difference in activity is the more remarkable when it is appreciated that the only difference in structure between the two chemicals is a single hydroxyl (OH) group.

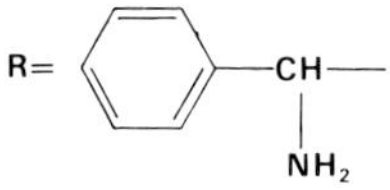

Ampicillin
side chain
                                               Amoxycillin 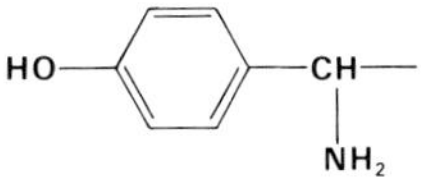
side chain

Because of their wide activity, both penicillins have activity against many of the organisms which can cause serious disease in animals.

A wide range of bacterial infections can be treated with both ampicillin and amoxycillin. These antibiotics are formulated in different ways suitable for application in various species of animals: as tablets, powders, cream and injectable formulations.

Carbenicillin

Carbenicillin was the first penicillin to have activity against *Pseudomonas aeruginosa*, an organism which, although ubiquitous, tends to become pathogenic to human beings and animals in the presence of existing infections such as chronic wounds, nephritis and chronic staphylococcal mastitis or when resistance is lowered because of some chronic infection. It is often difficult to eradicate the organism and high levels of drug need to be maintained at the site of infection if a cure is to be effected.

Carbenicillin is not stable in the presence of acid, so it has to be given by injection. Its use in animals is limited because of the relative infrequency with which a diagnosis of *Pseudomonas* infection is made and also because of the high levels of antibiotic which have to be maintained and the fact that it has to be injected rather than given orally. Its use, therefore, is confined to breeding stock, valuable horses and dogs.

Cephalosporins

The cephalosporins resemble penicillins in that they interfere with cell wall formation and thus have a bactericidal action and that their action covers a broad spectrum of organisms. Like penicillin, they originated from a fungus—in this case *Cephalosporium*—which was found in a sewage outflow in Sardinia.

They are based on a specific nucleus, 7-amino-cephalosporanic acid. The general structure is shown on p. 49 and new compounds are developed by substituting at points R_1 or R_2.

Although cephalosporins are used widely in human therapy, only a few have been developed for veterinary use. Most of them have a broad spectrum of activity, but some are unstable to β-lactamases produced by organisms such as staphylococci and *E coli*. Cephalothin, Cephaloridine, Cephoxazole, Cephalonium and Cefuroxime are all used in veterinary medicine but on a limited scale. This is not a reflection on their efficacy but rather on the fact that the penicillins were examined in much greater detail for animal therapy and at the time of their introduction were less expensive.

β-Lactamase inhibitors

β-Lactamase inhibitors cause irreversible inhibition of β-lactamase and prevent the enzyme attacking the susceptible -lactam ring in both penicillins and cephalosporins. They can now be combined with some penicillins such as amoxycillin to protect the penicillin from the attack of penicillinase-producing organisms.

One of the most active of the inhibitors, clavulanic acid, is itself a β-lactam and was obtained from *Streptomyces clavligerus*.

Clavulanic acid

Clavulanic acid combined with amoxycillin in a proportion of 1 to 4 is known in animal therapy as SYNULOX. With this preparation, an even release of both materials is obtained in the serum—this protects amoxycillin, and also reduces the level at which a normally resistant organism is sensitive to amoxycillin.

Tetracyclines

The discovery of the tetracycline range of chemicals followed the search that was initiated after the value of penicillin was established, to find sources of new antibiotics in the fungi which are found worldwide, particularly in areas of damp and decay. The first of a very active group of antibiotics was chlortetracycline, which was recovered from the actinomycete *Streptomyces aureofaciens* and was given the name Aureomycin. The name of the fungus was chosen because of the intense yellow colour of the cultures (Latin *aurum*—gold).

Chlortetracycline   Oxytetracycline

Chlortetracycline is extracted from fungal fermentation growth and is a yellow crystalline amphoteric compound. The structure of the group of compounds is based on the tetracycline nucleus and in the case of chlortetracycline, the hydrogen atom attached to carbon 7 is replaced by a chlorine atom.

Mode of action

The tetracyclines interfere with the bacterial protein synthesis in rapidly growing and reproducing bacterial cells. They inhibit the metabolism of the bacteria by blocking attachment of amino-acyl transfer ribonucleic acid ribosomes which interfere with complete protein synthesis. This action causes a bacteriostasis, which is due to inhibition of growth as the conversion of glutamate into cell protein by bacteria is slowed down.

Spectrum of activity

The tetracyclines are described as being broad-spectrum in action because they have a range of activity which covers the majority of Gram-positive and Gram-negative bacteria, and in addition they have activity against certain other sorts of pathogenic micro-organisms such as rickettsia and mycoplasms. Like penicillins, the tetracyclines are most active against rapidly growing organisms.

Chlortetracycline and the other tetracyclines since discovered (oxytetracycline, tetracycline, doxycycline, methacycline) have all found use in animal treatment. This is because of their wide spectrum of antibacterial activity and their persistence in the body.

Pharmacokinetics

Following oral administration they are readily absorbed from the stomach and small intestine. In young calves on a milk substitute diet, however, absorption may be reduced because of the tendency for tetracyclines to attach to the calcium ions. Unlike the penicillins, which reach a peak concentration in the plasma within half an hour, tetracyclines reach their peak more slowly, usually within 2 to 4 hours when given orally. They have, for animal treatment, the great additional advantage of persisting at high concentration in the serum for 6 hours and then at lower levels until the drug is finally no longer detectable at 24 hours. The tetracyclines diffuse well throughout the body and reach their highest concentrations in the kidney, liver and lung. They are removed from the blood by the liver and high levels are achieved in the bile. They are excreted mainly by the kidney but are also found in the faeces and milk.

Toxicology

Like the penicillins, the tetracyclines are relatively non-toxic.

They have some disadvantages, however.

(1) They can cause, when given orally, gastro-intestinal upsets in dogs, calves and horses.

(2) Both oxytetracycline and chlortetracycline can be irritant to the mammary tissue when given as a preventive therapy to the dry cow. In addition, chlortetracycline, in particular, cannot be given by the intramuscular or subcutaneous routes as it causes acute local irritation.

(3) All the tetracyclines are deposited in growing teeth and bones, so should not be given regularly to young growing animals.

Bacterial resistance

Resistance to members of the tetracycline group of antibiotics is frequently recorded following a course of treatment. Because of this their use as growth promoters in animal feeds has not been permitted since 1969 in the UK. It was considered that the ·risk of wide antibacterial resistance in animal populations would reduce their value in both animal and human treatments.

Aminoglycosides

The aminoglycoside antibiotics are composed of aminosugars connected by glycosidic linkages. They all have very similar antibacterial properties and also tend to show the same toxic effects. Many of the aminoglycosides were first developed for human usage and later found a place in animal treatment. The most important ones are streptomycin and dihydrostreptomycin, neomycin and gentamicin.

Mode of action

The aminoglycosides are bactericidal and act on the 30s ribosomal sub-unit to stop the synthesis of bacterial cell protein.

Spectrum of activity

The aminoglycosides have a more limited range of activity than either the penicillins or the tetracyclines and they are mainly used clinically against Gram-negative organisms. Some have activity against Gram-positive organisms but the activity is usually of a lower order than the penicillins or tetracyclines.

As the aminoglycosides tend to be considered as separate entities, they are here given individual consideration.

Streptomycin and dihydrostreptomycin

Streptomycin was the first new antibiotic from a fungal source to be described following the successful use of penicillin. It was reported in 1944 following its isolation from a mould, *Streptomyces griseus*, which was recovered from heavily manured soil near the farm buildings of the Rutgers University Agricultural Station in New Jersey.

It is active against a range of Gram-negative bacteria such as *Pasteurella*, *Brucella*, *Haemophilus*, *Salmonella*, *Klebsiella*, *Shigella* and *Mycobacterium*. This Gram-negative activity makes it complementary in action to penicillin and in the animal treatment field combinations of penicillin and streptomycin are still in common use. One of its most exciting and unique activities is that against the tubercle bacillus, the cause of tuberculosis in humans. Professor S. A. Waksman, one of the discoverers of the antibiotic, was awarded the Nobel prize for medicine in 1952 because of the importance of this finding.

Dihydrostreptomycin was produced two years after the discovery of streptomycin and it was hoped that it would be less toxic than the parent compound, but it was eventually found to have similar neurotoxic action to that found with streptomycin.

Streptomycin   Dihydrostreptomycin

Pharmacokinetics

Neither streptomycin nor dihydrostreptomycin is absorbed across the intestinal mucosa when given orally so that for general use they must be given by injection. Following intramuscular injection, streptomycin reaches maximum plasma levels within 60 minutes. Adequate concentrations of antibiotic are found in the fluids of body cavities and the drug also diffuses into the foetal blood and placenta. It is found in the milk and this is of value in the treatment of mastitis in dairy cattle.

Streptomycin is excreted primarily in the urine, about two thirds of an intramuscular dose being cleared within 24 hours. In some cases, however, where large doses of dihydrostreptomycin have been given, a residue may be detected in the kidneys as long as 90 days after dosing. This type of residue poses serious problems if the animals are to be consumed within this time.

Toxicology

The most important feature associated with the use of the streptomycins is their action on the vestibules and auditory mechanisms which are supplied by the 8th cranial nerve. Toxic symptoms following treatment were first recognized in the cat and dog, probably because owners recognize the abnormal gait caused by chronic nerve damage. Neurotoxic damage is less likely to be recognized in the cow or pig as these animals are not observed in the same detail. Neurotoxic effects can influence posture and gait and continual administration can lead to permanent damage to the vestibular organ in the ear.

If the correct therapeutic dose is adhered to in animals, however, the risk of neurotoxicity is low.

Bacterial resistance

Streptomycin therapy can lead to a marked increase in resistant bacteria even during the course of therapy. It is important, therefore, when using the streptomycins to monitor the effect of therapy very carefully, so that if no response to treatment is noticed within two to three days, the use of either streptomycin or dihydrostreptomycin is discontinued. Bacteria which are resistant to streptomycin are also resistant to dihydrostreptomycin and some other aminoglycosides.

Neomycin

Neomycin was isolated from an actinomycete which was found in a soil sample from the farmyard of Rutgers University where streptomycin was found earlier. The source organism in this case was *Streptomyces fradiae*. This antibiotic was reported seven years after the discovery of streptomycin. It has a very similar range of action to that of streptomycin. In veterinary medicine its major uses are as a topical preparation for skin and ear infections, and orally for enteritis in calves and pigs due to coliform organisms. Like the streptomycins it can cause damage to both the auditory nerve and the kidneys, so that it is little used parenterally and the main dosage forms are either tablets or powders to be given by the oral route or creams to be given by the topical route for skin or ear infections.

Pharmacokinetics

Neomycin is absorbed to the extent of about 3% when given orally, so that it can be given with confidence for gut infections by the oral route and when dosed in this way, most of the drug is excreted unchanged in the faeces.

Toxicology

Although neomycin can cause irreversible damage to the auditory division of the 8th cranial nerve if given by injection, treatment of the skin or oral therapy are unlikely to lead to any observable toxic effects.

Bacterial resistance

Resistance to neomycin has been recognized following oral therapy of both calves and pigs, but resistant strains seldom dominate in the bacterial flora.

Gentamicin

Gentamicin was reported some 20 years after the discovery of strepto-mycin—it was obtained from a fungus called *Micromonospora purpurea*. Gentamicin is more active than the earlier aminoglycosides against many Gram-negative organisms and is used both topically and by the intra-muscular route. In the human clinical field its activity is particularly out-standing against *Pseudomonas* species, and it is also used in life-threatening infections before a bacteriological diagnosis has been made because of its known high activity.

Gentamicin has been used in poultry in a variety of ways.
(1) Fertile turkey eggs are dipped in a solution of gentamicin to reduce the possibility of *Mycoplasma* infection in newly born poults.
(2) Turkey poults can be treated to control gut infections and prevent the young bird becoming a carrier of *Salmonella arizona* infections.
(3) Gentamicin is also used in dogs and cats to treat urinary and respiratory infections which are not responding to other antibacterial treatment.

Pharmacokinetics

As with other aminoglycosides, gentamicin is poorly absorbed when given orally, but when given by the intramuscular route it is absorbed rapidly and produces peak serum concentrations 30–60 minutes after administration.

Toxicology

As with other aminoglycosides, gentamicin therapy can cause damage to the vestibular functions of the 8th cranial nerve. This is most likely to occur when there is impaired renal function. It is usual, therefore, to use gentamicin in cats and dogs only when other forms of therapy have failed.

Bacterial resistance

Resistance can develop and, should this occur, the bacteria will in many cases be resistant to other aminoglycosides.

Macrolide antibiotics

Macrolide antibiotics contain a large lactone ring with sugars attached. The principal macrolide used for animal treatment is tylosin, which was first isolated from *Streptomyces fradiae*, found in soil in Thailand.

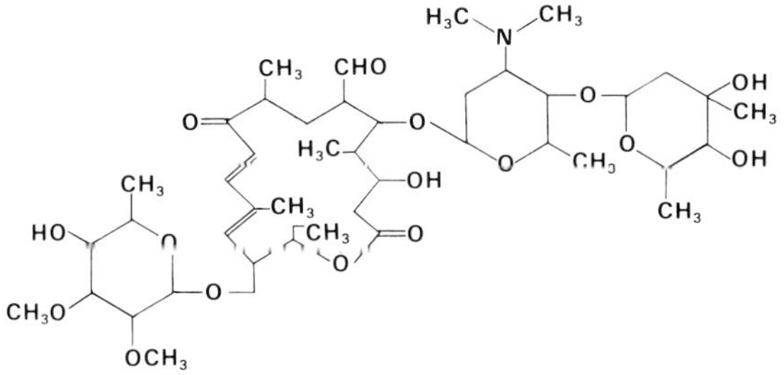

Tylosin

   Macrolides are active against Gram-positive organisms and were first used against those which were resistant to penicillin.

Mode of action

The macrolide antibiotics act by interfering with the normal development of the protein combinations necessary for bacterial growth. They influence, in particular, the process of translocation—the movement of an aminoglycoside to a donor site on the ribosome is prevented.

Spectrum of activity

There are a number of macrolides which are used for the treatment and prevention of animal disease: tylosin, erythromycin, oleandomycin and spiramycin. Tylosin is the outstanding macrolide in the animal field. The other three macrolides are used for animal therapy to a certain extent, but their activities have not shown any special characteristics which would merit their wide use. Tylosin was introduced in 1962 as an antibiotic specifically for use in animals and is still in use in all major animal-producing areas as a feed additive growth promoter which is included in poultry and pig feeds. This aspect of its use will be mentioned later in the chapter on growth promotion.

In addition to its activity against Gram-positive bacteria, it has antimycoplasma and antitreponema properties. It is this combination of action against Gram-positive organisms, *Mycoplasma* and *Treponema hyodysenteria* which has made it particularly valuable for use in pigs.

Pharmacokinetics

Tylosin as the tartrate salt is well absorbed when given orally and achieves a maximum blood concentration one hour after administration. It is excreted in the urine and bile.

Toxicology

Toxicity studies have shown that tylosin has a wide margin of safety in all species of animals.

Antibiotics of miscellaneous structure

Tiamulin

Tiamulin is a derivative of pleuromutilin, an active antibiotic obtained from the mould *Pleurotus mutilis*. It is used clinically and has been developed as a growth promoter with specific action against Gram-positive organisms, *Mycoplasma* and *Treponema hyodysenteria*. It is used in pigs and poultry for the control of respiratory infections and in pigs for the control of swine dysentery.

Mode of action

Tiamulin acts as an inhibitor of protein synthesis and thus prevents the development of the bacterial cell.

Pharmacokinetics

Tiamulin is well absorbed by the oral route and is converted into active metabolites which accumulate in the tissues, particularly in the respiratory system. This allows prolonged antibacterial and antimycoplasma action.

Toxicology

The only significant toxic risk is related to its use in poultry in association with the anticoccidiostat monensin (see chapter 8). Tiamulin interferes with monensin metabolism and this can lead to toxic reactions in poultry.

Lincomycin

Lincomycin was discovered from a soil sample taken in Lincoln, Nebraska, which yielded *Streptomyces lincolnensis*. Its antibacterial spectrum is similar to that of the macrolides. Lincomycin accumulates in certain tissues, such as skin and lungs, which enhances its value for the treatment of infections in these areas.

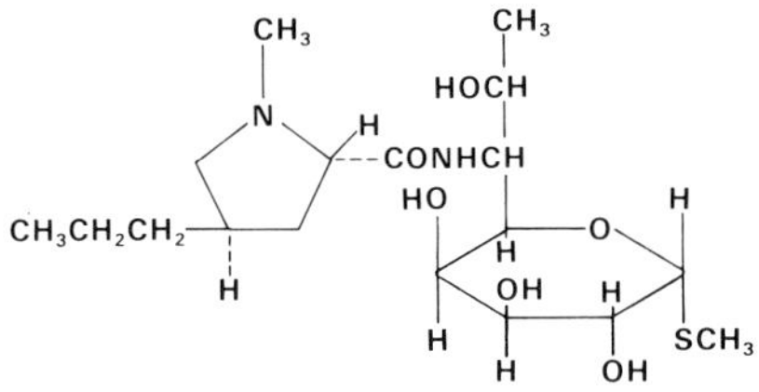

Lincomycin

Mode of action

Lincomycin acts by interfering with protein synthesis, particularly with the process of translocation in the bacterial cell. It is well absorbed when given by mouth, and is active for 6–8 hours in the blood. It is distributed widely throughout the body. In dogs, when the drug is given orally, 77% of the drug is excreted in the faeces.

Resistance

Lincomycin shows a cross-resistance to macrolide antibiotics.

Mupirocin

Mupirocin is a naturally occurring compound which is produced by the mould *Pseudomonas fluorescens*.

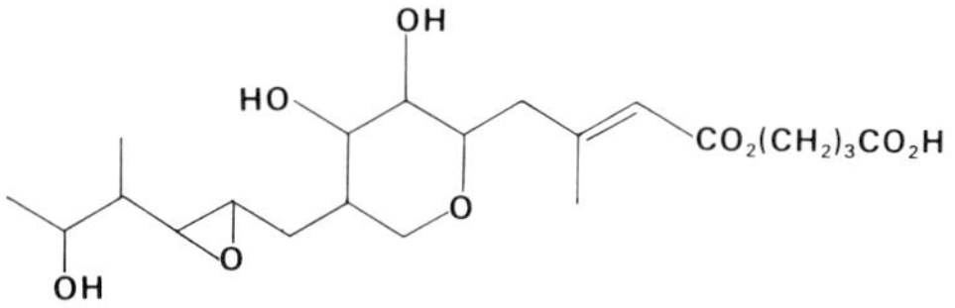

Mupirocin

It is principally active against Gram-positive bacteria such as staphylococci and streptococci. It is also active against some Gram-negative species such as *Haemophilus*, *Pasteurella* and *Bordetella*, and against *Treponema* and *Mycoplasma*.

Mupirocin is active as a growth promoter in pigs as the calcium salt dihydrate.

Mode of action

Mupirocin prevents protein synthesis by binding with the enzyme isoleucyl transfer RNA synthetase. It is absorbed through the gut and is rapidly and completely metabolized to inactive monic acid by splitting off the carbon side chain.

6. Anthelmintics

Introduction

When one considers the wide range of helminth parasites found in animals, it is not surprising that anthelmintics are high on the list of chemicals used for animal disease control. The way of life of both farm and domestic animals provides the environment necessary for continuity of all the major helminth species. Farm animals, and cattle and sheep in particular, depend for their existence in most parts of the world on the grazing of pastures, and they may eat extraneous material that can be found on the ground. In addition, they continually return to graze on areas which have been contaminated by their own faeces or that of their companions. The eggs or larval stages of the majority of the helminths are passed in the faeces and depend for their future development on being taken in again by mouth. Many schemes have been evolved for parasite control which involve the movement of animals on to clean pastures at regular intervals to prevent re-infestation with the eggs or larvae of helminths, but they are seldom practised by the farmer as they require both careful planning and a fairly large area of grazing.

Domestic animals such as cats and dogs, particularly in towns, pick up their infestations from the faeces-contaminated streets and pavements, while in the country they propagate infestations by eating the liver or lungs of secondary helminth hosts which contain larval stages. Examples of such hosts are rabbits and mice. In addition, they carry their own re-infesters, as the dog flea acts as intermediate host for the larval stage of a major tapeworm found in dogs.

Helminth researchers over the last 30 years have described the pattern of the life cycles of the majority of helminth parasites in animals. This has helped in the drawing up of control programmes for the more important parasites, and these programmes are now recommended to farmers and to dog and horse owners.

The programmes will involve:

(1) courses of treatment with anthelmintics at strategic times in the life cycle of important parasites, for example, (a) at the recognized hatching period of larvae on the ground, (b) when liver fluke larvae first appear in the liver of

infested sheep, (c) when infested adults are most likely to pass on their infection to susceptible young animals;

(2) the maintainance of pastures free of sheep or cattle, so that uninfected lambs or calves can have their initial grazing experience on those pastures free from the danger of picking up worm larvae;

(3) the thorough cleaning of premises for housed animals before introduction of uninfected cats, dogs or piglets;

(4) advice on the treatment of bitches and puppies for ascarid infestations to prevent spread from bitch to puppy, and to reduce the danger of larval spread from infested dog to human beings.

It has always to be remembered that the use of an anthelmintic alone is often inadequate as a means of completely eliminating a parasite infestation, as the majority of anthelmintics are present in the body for only a few hours, so that re-infestation from a contaminated area can occur within 24 hours of treatment.

Types of helminth or worm found in animals

There are three major types of helminth—tapeworms (Figure 6.1), flukes (Figure 6.2) and roundworms (Figure 6.3). Tapeworms are flat and segmented, and are found mainly in the intestines. Liver flukes are also flat, but oval shaped, and are found in the liver of sheep and cattle. Roundworms are the major parasites of all animals and vary in size from less than 7 mm to 30 cm. In the adult form they live mainly in the stomach and intestines but can be found in many parts of the body during larval migration.

Clinical and pathological effects of helminths on their host

Helminths produce different symptoms and lesions in their hosts according to the site of their major area of action (Table 6.1). Some of their habitats are described below:

The *tapeworm* lives in the small intestine and depends for its survival on absorbing nutrients from the host's food, so that of itself it does little physical damage.

The *hookworm*—a variety of roundworm found in cattle, sheep, dogs and cats—lives by sucking blood whilst attached to the intestinal wall of its host. This leads to loss of weight and retarded growth and often physical weakness.

The *redworm* is a roundworm which lives in the intestine of the horse and feeds on the host's tissues, leading to loss of racing form and, in some cases, emaciation.

The *ascarids* are a group of large roundworms which are found particularly in the horse, pig, dog and cat and can cause mechanical obstruction of

Table 6.1.   Common helminths found in domestic animals and their site of action.

Animal	Roundworms	Flukes	Tapeworms
Cattle and sheep	Stomach and intestines Lungs	Liver	Intestines
Pig	Stomach and intestines Lungs	—	Intestines
Horse	Intestines Lungs	—	—
Dog	Intestines Heart and arteries	—	Intestines
Cat	Intestines	—	Intestines
Poultry	Intestines Trachea	—	Intestines

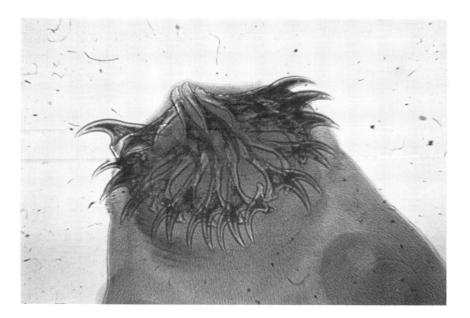

Figure 6.1 (*a*) Head of *Taenia*.

the gut because of their numbers and size. They can provide a severe problem in the rearing of puppies, kittens and young pigs.

The heartworm is a small roundworm called *Dirofilaria immitis* which establishes itself in the circulatory system of the dog, principally in the right side of the heart in the pulmonary artery although it is also found in the posterior vena cava. It can cause pneumonitis, and in more severe cases it will lead to thrombus formation as a result of damage to the cells of the vascular

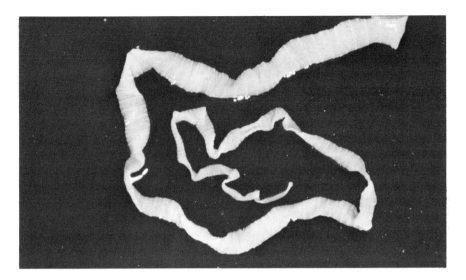

Figure 6.1 (*b*) *Taenia hydatigena*. Tapeworm of the dog (up to 5 m long).

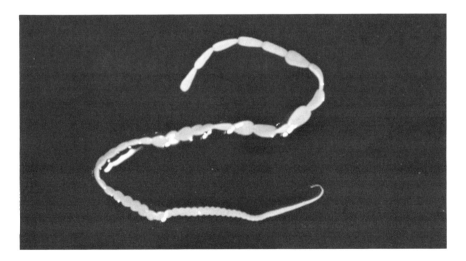

Figure 6.1 (*c*) *Dipylidium caninum*. Tapeworm of dog (up to 75 cm long).

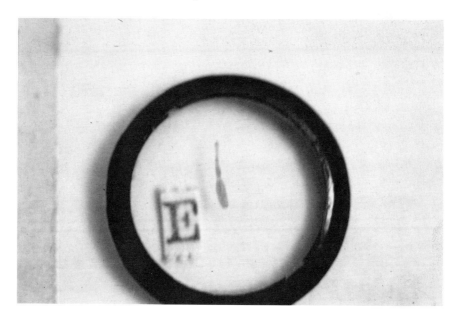

Figure 6.1 (*d*) *Echinococcus granulosus*. Tapeworm of the dog (up to 9 mm long).

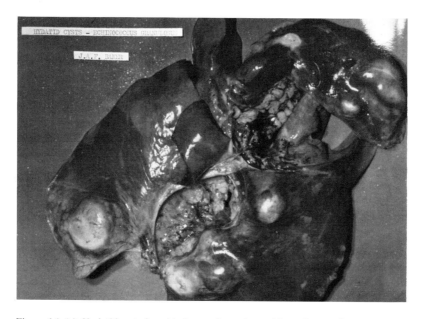

Figure 6.1 (*e*) Hydatid cysts found in human lungs (up to 10 cm diameter).

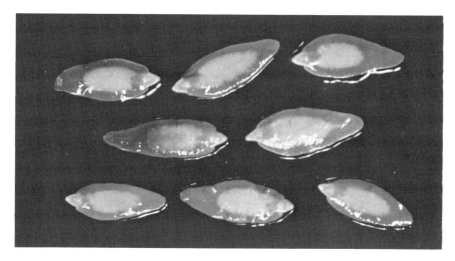

Figure 6.2.   *Fasciola hepatica*. The major liver fluke of the sheep (5 cm long, 1·5 cm wide).

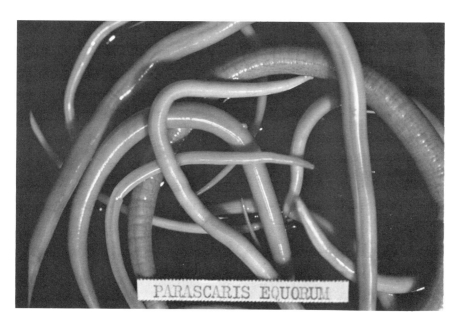

Figure 6.3.   Roundworms
(*a*) *Parascaris equorum*. The large roundworm of the horse (males up to 28 cm long, females
     50 cm).

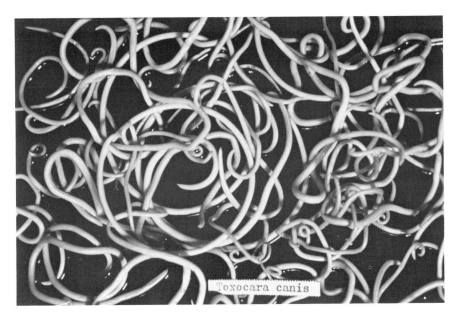

Figure 6.3 (*b*) *Toxocara cants*. The major roundworm of the dog (males up to 10 cm long, females 18 cm).

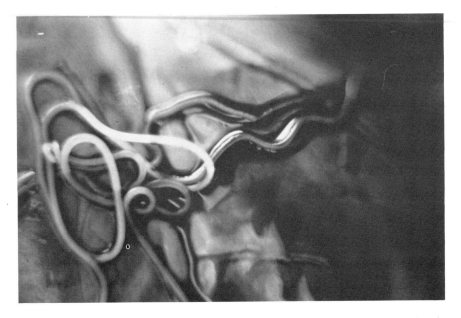

Figure 6.3 (*c*) *Dirofilaria*. Larval stage of the heartworm of the dog (males up to 8 cm, females 10 cm).

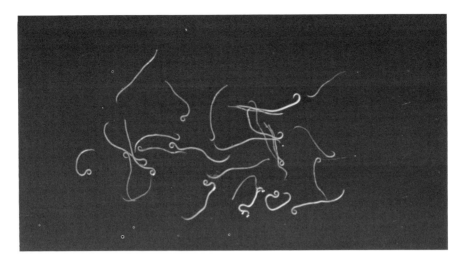

Figure 6.3 (*d*) *Oesophagostomum radiatum.*

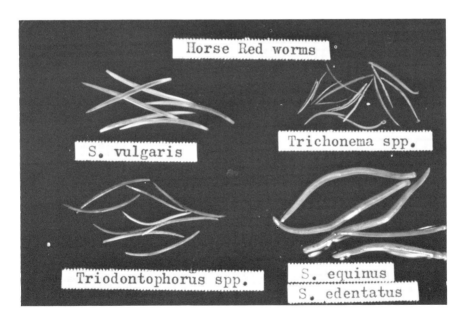

Figure 6.3 (*e*) Various horse roundworms.

system. The larval stage of this helminth is transmitted by the bite of the mosquito so that infestations are seen mainly in the warmer parts of the world such as the southern USA, South America and Australia and the Mediterranean countries.

The significance of helminth infestations

Helminth parasites can appear in many parts of the body of an animal, and their relevance will depend on the standards of control practised in an animal community, be it small or large. For instance, the helminth problem encountered by the individual hill sheep in Scotland will be of a different degree to that experienced by an individual member of the flocks of up to 60 000 sheep kept in Australia or Argentina. The efficacy of an anthelmintic drug in therapy will be greatly influenced by the state of infestation of an animal or flock at the time of treatment, by the number of animals in the environment and by the possibility of preventing re-infestation after treatment. The aim of treatment is to eliminate the existing infestation, but even if achieved the effect may be minimized by the relatively short period of activity of an anthelmintic within the animal. Ideally, after treatment animals should be moved to parasite-free pastures or clean accommodation so that no new infestation develops.

Where farm animals are permanently at pasture or dogs and cats are kept in the confined area of kennels (where the survival of the parasites is favoured), heavy parasite infestations can occur. If, in addition, external factors such as climatic conditions suit the parasites, continual infestations are likely to be maintained within the animals. In such circumstances, regular treatment with an anthelmintic may well be necessary if the worm burden is to be kept at a low level. It is important, however, to remember that some parasite exposure is necessary if immunity to the parasite is to be developed.

The excessive use of one anthelmintic in an environment can also lead to the dominance of resistant strains of helminths. This is most likely to happen in large flocks where frequent treatment may have to be carried out because of permanent heavy pasture contamination. As in so many other spheres of disease due to infectious agents, efficient therapy depends on the user understanding the relationship between the biology and environment of the parasite and the strategy of anthelmintic treatment.

To assist helminth control many new anthelmintics have been developed which are both host-specific and highly effective against both the adult and larval stages of parasites.

Mode of action of anthelmintics

The anthelmintics used to treat animals in the 1930s were selected largely because they appeared to reduce parasite infestations without at the same time killing the host. Many of the chemicals used at that time, however, were only marginally safe and their use had often to be followed by treatment with either an antidote or a purgative to ensure elimination. Such chemicals as copper sulphate, arsenic compounds, nicotine and carbon tetrachloride, and herbal remedies such as oil of chenopodium, extract of male fern, santonin and quassia, were all used as anthelmintics. Apart from having a narrow therapeutic index (meaning that the therapeutic dose is very close to the toxic level), the majority of these chemicals acted as irritants leading to increased bowel motility rather than having a specific action on the individual helminths.

During the last ten years, in order to develop a better understanding of the anthelmintic action of new chemicals, investigations have been carried out into the biochemical and physiological functions of individual helminth species, and this has helped in the search for new anthelmintics with highly specific action. Because helminths possess muscle and nervous systems, and primitive circulatory and excretory systems which can be affected by active anthelmintics, detailed study in the laboratory of the effect of exposure of a worm to an anthelmintic has allowed the mode of action of many of the newer anthelmintics to be established. These modes of action can be considered under two main headings, depending on whether they involve disruption of energy metabolism or of neuromuscular action.

Effect on energy metabolism

Anthelmintics can influence the energy metabolism of parasites in a number of ways:
(1) inhibition of glucose transport—glucose has to be converted into glycogen (a soluble starch) for storage;
(2) disruption of glycogen metabolism;
(3) inhibition of glycolysis (the first stage in the conversion of glucose by enzyme action into lactic acid);
(4) inhibition of mitochondrial reactions which lead to inhibition of fumarate reduction enzyme activity and then to blocking of the generation of energy bonds and eventual muscular paralysis and death of the parasite; action on mitochondria interferes with DNA;
(5) uncoupling of electron transport.

Effect on the neuromuscular system

(1) Inhibitory effect of organophosphorus drugs on the enzyme acetylcholinesterase.
(2) A curare-like effect which leads to paralysis of the worm and its eventual expulsion.
(3) Cholinergic agonists acting at the ganglion level.

Characteristics of a good anthelmintic

An ideal anthelmintic would have at least the five following characteristics.
(1) It should have a wide therapeutic index, so that animals can be dosed with safety. This is particularly important in the case of sheep and cattle which may have been mustered from a large area for dosing, are often in a poor state at the time of treatment and may not be seen again for several weeks after dosing.
(2) It should have a broad spectrum of activity against all worm forms in the animal at the time of treatment, including both larval and adult stages.
(3) It should be simple to administer and, if possible, palatable.
(4) It should be economic to use.
(5) It should have a short residual period in the tissues, so that there are no significant residue problems after treatment.

Formulations of anthelmintics

The methods of presentation of anthelmintics have been continually adapted to suit the changes in management of domestic animals. The aim has always been to ensure that every animal gets an even and safe dose at the time of treatment. Where individual animals are to be treated, especially in the case of dogs, cats and horses, palatability is often a very important factor, whereas when thousands of sheep and cattle have to be collected and treated in one day, speed and ease of administration is of paramount importance.

Suspensions and solutions are particularly suitable for use with a dosing gun. Suspensions have to be well shaken before use to ensure even dosing.

Injectable preparations can be used safely only when the chemical has been proven to be non-irritant and to disperse readily from the site of injection. Suitable drugs are levamisole, ivermectin, diethyl carbamazine.

Pour-on preparations depend on the fact that the active principle when applied as a liquid to the skin is rapidly absorbed, as happens with, for example, levamisole.

Preparations which can be added to the feed are usually prepared in the form of cubes or small pellets which can be incorporated in the normal feed of the treated animals. The whole dose should be mixed in the feed and given in the morning. Adequate trough space must be available so that each animal can ingest the full dose.

Resistance to anthelmintics

Only in the last few years has it been considered likely that the use of anthelmintics would lead to the development of important resistance problems. Reports of serious occurrence of resistance, particularly to the benzimidazole group of chemicals, have come from Australia, where anthelmintics are used probably more widely than in any other animal-rearing country.

The resistance in the case of benzimidazole is considered to be carried by one gene, so that very frequent use of one such anthelmintic can lead to the build-up of helminth resistance quite rapidly, particularly if the same anthelmintic is used all the time. The likelihood of resistance occurring in Australia is due in large measure to the fact that there may be four or more parasite cycles in one year compared with one or two cycles in Europe. This is due to both the high temperature and heavy rains commonly encountered in the sheep pastures.

It is now recommended that to reduce the risk of a resistance problem following treatment, drugs should be alternated on sheep properties where frequent treatments have to take place. When a new anthelmintic is introduced it should belong to a chemical group different from that previously used on the property. Resistance in helminths appears to be a problem of therapy mainly in sheep, as these animals receive the most frequent treatment and up to 50 000 sheep may be treated regularly on one property. In some ways the occurrence of anthelmintic resistance on a large sheep farm has a resemblance to the appearance of bacterial resistance in some of the wards of hospitals where a specific bacterial infection is frequently present. In the one case all the animals are treated regularly with the same anthelmintic, and in the hospital all the patients receive the same antibiotic therapy, often for long periods. In both these cases the apparent advantages of a closed community are vitiated by the tendency to also maintain a highly selected bacterial or parasite population.

Causes of variation in activity of anthelmintics

Apart from the obvious inefficiency of using an anthelmintic on an already-resistant worm population, there are a number of other factors which will affect the success of treatment.

(1) A proper diagnosis of the worm infestation to be treated must be made before therapy is begun, as such symptoms as poor growth, loss of appetite, diarrhoea and coughing in animals can often be due to causes other than worms.

(2) Inefficient methods of dosing of a large group of animals can lead to too high or too low a dose of anthelmintic being given to individual animals. This

type of failure can often be corrected by testing the calibration of a dosing gun before treatment commences.

(3) The right anthelmintic must be used for the specific infestation present in the animals to be treated.

(4) Certain specific anthelmintics are effective against both adult and larval stages of worms, and only these should be used in both sheep and cattle if effective control is to be achieved.

Anthelmintics in general use for animal treatment

Because of the range of helminths and their sites of action in animals, a wide variety of chemical structures have been investigated for anthelmintic activity and subsequently prepared for animal treatment. It is possible to classify anthelmintics under a number of headings and Tables 6.2 to 6.5 show the range of activity of the main chemicals used in cattle and sheep, dogs and cats, horses and pigs.

Benzimidazoles

The benzimidazoles form a very active group of chemicals which have played the predominant part in the control of worm infestations in sheep, cattle and horses since the introduction of the first of the group, thiabendazole, in 1961. It was followed by parbendazole in 1967, but it was cambendazole, introduced in 1970, which significantly extended the activity of the series by showing activity against the larval stages of worms found in the intestines. Previously, larval stages had resisted treatment so that an initial response to therapy was often followed by a new outbreak of helminthiasis when larval stages moulted and attached to the gut wall as adults.

Cambendazole was followed by mebendazole (1971), oxibendazole (1973), fenbendazole (1974), oxfendazole (1975) and albendazole (1976).

Table 6.6 gives the chemical structures of the different benzimidazoles.

Mode of action

The benzimidazoles produce their effect on helminths by influencing the uptake of nutrients. They affect the activity of the enzyme fumarate reductase, which leads to a reduction in glycogen and starvation of the helminth. It seems probable that this effect is enhanced by the prolonged period of activity of the drug associated with low solubility. For instance, albendazole and fenbendazole may take up to 24 hours to reach peak level in the blood.

Table 6.2. Main anthelmintics used in sheep and cattle.

| Chemicals | Types of worms or activity | | | |
	Gastro-intestinal	Lung	Tapeworms	Liver fluke
BROAD SPECTRUM				
Benzimidazoles	+	+	±	±
Tetrahydro-imidazothiazoles	+	+	−	−
Avermectins	+	+	−	−
NARROW SPECTRUM				
Tetrahydro-pyrimidines	+	−	−	−
Organophosphorus compounds	+	−	−	−
Anilidines and substituted phenols	±	−	±	±

+ High activity against the majority of adult and larval stages of worms.
− Inactive.
± Some anthelmintics in the class are active against all worms described, whereas others have positive activity against major worms and none against other species.

Table 6.3. Main anthelmintics used in dogs and cats.

| Chemicals | Types of worms | | | | Tapeworms |
| | Roundworms | | | | |
	Large roundworms	Hookworms	Whipworms	Heartworms	
BROAD SPECTRUM					
Mebendazole	++	++	++	−	++
Nitroscanate	++	++	−	−	++
Dichlorovos	++	++	++	−	−
NARROW SPECTRUM					
Bunamidine	−	−	−	−	++
Praziquantel	−	−	−	−	++
Piperazine salts	+	+	−	−	−
Diethyl carbamazine	+	−	−	+	−

++ High activity.
+ Acceptable activity.
− Inactive.

Spectrum of action

The benzimidazoles remove the major adult stomach and intestinal roundworms to the extent of 85–100%. Albendazole, fenbendazole and oxfendazole are also active against liver fluke and tapeworms in addition to their roundworm activity. This has meant that this remarkable range of

Table 6.4.   Main anthelmintics used in horses.

| | Roundworms | |
Chemical	Strongyles	Ascarids
BROAD SPECTRUM		
Benzimidazoles*	+	+
Levamisole	+	+
Dichlorvos	+	+
Avermectins	+	+
Piperazines	±	+

* Substituted benzimidazoles most active, e.g., mebendazole.
+ Acceptable activity.
± Some anthelmintics in the class are active against all worms
  described, whereas others have positive activity against
  major worms and none against other species.

Table 6.5.   Main anthelmintics used in pigs.

| | Roundworms | | |
Chemical	Strongyles	Ascarids	Lungworm
Benzimidazoles*	+	+	+ *
Levamisole	+	+	+
Dichlorvos	±	+	±
Piperazines	±	+	−
Avermectins	+	+	+

* Oxfendazole most active.
+ Acceptable activity.
− Inactive.
± Some anthelmintics in the class are active against all worms described, whereas
  others have positive activity against major worms and none against other species.

anthelmintics has paid a key part in improving the efficiency of treatment of
cattle, sheep, horses and pigs. Mebendazole is also of considerable value as a
broad-spectrum treatment in dogs and cats.

Pharmacokinetics

Thiabendazole, the first of the group, is readily absorbed after oral administration and is distributed throughout the body. It reaches its peak concentration in blood after 4 hours. It is metabolized by hydroxylation at the 5-
position, followed by conjugation with glucuronic acid or sulphate. About
90% of a dose is excreted by treated animals in the urine and 5% in the faeces
in 48 hours. The major portion is excreted as conjugated 5-hydroxy-
thiabendazole.

Table 6.6.   Representative structures of benimidazoles.

Thiabendazole	
Parbendazole	
Cambendazole	
Mebendazole	
Oxibendazole	
Fenbendazole	
Albendazole	
Oxfendazole	

The newer benzimidazoles, by contrast, are metabolized and excreted much more slowly. This is achieved by blocking the 5-position. Another group is substituted in the 5-position and the thiazole ring is replaced by methyl carbamate. This change causes slower elimination and leads to greater activity at lower dose levels and an increase in the spectrum of activity, particularly against larval stages.

Table 6.7.   Dose levels of benzimidazoles in sheep and cattle.

	Dose (mg/kg bodyweight)
Thiabendazole	66
Parbendazole	20
Cambendazole	25
Oxibendazole	10
Mebendazole	15
Albendazole	7·5
Fenbendazole	7·5
Oxfendazole	4·5

The effect of this change on dosage levels in sheep and cattle is evident in the figures shown in Table 6.7.

Toxicology

The majority of the benzimidazoles are well tolerated at therapeutic levels by animals and can be given with safety. Cambendazole is the only member of the group which has shown toxic reactions near the therapeutic dose. This is associated with inappetence and listlessness.

Where higher doses of albendazole are given to treat liver fluke in sheep, a teratogenic effect has been noted. To avoid this, ewes should not be treated for liver fluke infestations at mating time or for a month after conception.

Tetrahydro-imidathiazoles and tetrahydro-pyrimidines

The first of the tetrahydro-imidathiazoles, tetramisole, was a racemic mixture of two optical isomers and when it became possible to separate the isomers it was found that the anthelmintic activity rested mainly in the *l*-isomer, levamisole. Levamisole therefore became the drug of choice.

Morantel, a tetrahydro-pyrimidine, has an activity which is confined to the stomach and intestinal roundworms.

Mode of action

Levamisole has a paralysing effect on nematodes. It acts as a ganglion stimulant which leads to a sustained muscular contraction. At very high concentration the drug can inhibit fumarate reductase, but the main effect is paralysis of the nematode and its rejection.

Morantel acts as a neuromuscular blocking agent having a paralysing effect on the nematodes.

Table 6.8. Structures and dose levels of levamisole, tetramisole and morantel.

Name	Structure	Usual dose (mg/kg bodyweight)
Levamisole		7·5
Tetramisole		15
Morantel		8·8 in cattle 10 in sheep

Field usage

Levamisole has proved to be a very effective anthelmintic against the stomach, intestinal and lungworms of sheep and cattle. It is usually given either by mouth or subcutaneous injection. In addition, it can be given by 'pour on' for absorption through the skin of cattle.

Morantel is given by mouth and its activity in both sheep and cattle is limited by a lack of activity against the lungworms. It is now used in the form of a specially developed slow-release bolus which is given to cattle at the start of the grazing season. Pyrantel embonate, a pyrimidine related to morantel, is used for the treatment of roundworm infestations in the horse.

Pharmacokinetics

Levamisole is rapidly absorbed from the gut and carried to all parts of the body. When given by injection, peak blood levels are reached within an hour. It is excreted in the urine (40% within 12 hours) and up to 41% of the dose is excreted via the faeces. Tissue residues are not significant but in the USA a seven-day slaughter clearance has been decreed.

Morantel and pyrantel have similar pharmacological patterns and the drugs are well absorbed from the gut and achieve significant blood levels within 4 hours. They are quickly metabolized, 25% is excreted in the urine and the remainder passes out unchanged in the faeces.

Toxicology

Although levamisole has a narrower safety range than the benzimidazoles, the safety margin is about 12 times the dose so that reactions following treatment are unlikely. Because of the seven-day withholding time, treatment should not be given within seven days of slaughter. In the USA it is recommended that levamisole should not be given to animals of breeding age.

Morantel and pyrantel are safe for the animals for which they are normally prescribed (cattle, sheep and horses) and there is no significant residue problem.

Avermectins

The avermectins, first reported in 1979, constitute a new chemical class which offers activity against both a range of helminths and external parasites which are common pathogens of domestic animals.

This is the first effective anthelmintic derived from a fungal growth. The active principle was first recovered from the fermentation broth of actinomycete cultures received from Japan. The most active actinomycete was *Streptomyces avermitilis*, one of over 40 000 actinomycete cultures tested. The original culture was treated with ultraviolet light to generate mutants which would give higher yields of the active principle, avermectin.

The isolated avermectins contain a mixture of related chemical substances. The most effective anthelmintic is obtained by hydrogenation of the main extract to yield a product called ivermectin. This contains 80% of the 22,23-dihydroavermectin shown here and 20% of the corresponding substance with an isopropyl group at the 25-position.

22,23-dihydroavermectin B_{1a}

Mode of action

Ivermectin acts in the worm by blocking signal transmission from inter-neurons to excitatory motoneurons and GABA (γ-amino-butyric acid) is the neurotransmitter that is blocked. Its action is therefore as a GABA agonist.

Spectrum of activity

Ivermectin is highly active against nematodes and arthropods (insects, ticks and mites). It has a broad spectrum against the major nematodes of domestic animals but is inactive against tapeworms and liver fluke.

The most notable feature of the activity of ivermectin is its high potency when compared with any other anthelmintic. This is shown by its activity against the lungworm *Dictyocaulus vivipara* in cattle at 0·05 mg/kg bodyweight when given orally, compared with 7·5 mg/kg for levamisole and 5 mg/kg for fenbendazole. The standard dose for sheep, cattle and horses is 0·2 mg/kg and for pigs 0·3 mg/kg.

It will be seen that this anthelmintic is a real advance in the treatment of nematodes in domestic animals. It has been tested at single monthly doses for the prevention of establishment of heartworm in dogs with promising results.

The spectrum of activity against external parasites will be discussed in Chapter 7.

Pharmacokinetics

Little has been published on the pharmacology of ivermectin in animals, but Pritchard *et al.* (1985) reported on the behaviour of the drug in sheep when given intravenously and directly into the abomasum and rumen. They found that when given intravenously, ivermectin was slowly eliminated with a terminal half-life of 175 hours, whereas intra-abomasal administration resulted in rapid absorption with a peak plasma concentration of 60·6 mg/ml at 4·4 hours. Intraruminal administration produced a lower peak of 17·6 mg/ml at 23·5 hours. The long half-life of ivermectin reported when the drug is given intravenously would explain the high efficiency when the drug is given subcutaneously. It seems that a high proportion of active principle is distributed to extravascular tissues such as lipids and liver, so that storage takes place. Long half-life with anthelmintics has been found to influence potency.

Toxicology

The fact that ivermectin acts on GABA-mediated nerves means that the drug is unlikely to have a significant effect on mammalian tissue as GABA-mediated effect occurs only in the central nervous system in mammals.

Studies in rats have shown that little ivermectin crosses the blood–brain barrier. Other tests have shown that there is a considerable safety margin using the recommended dose.

There is a 14-day withholding period for treated animals and the drug is not recommended for lactating cattle.

Organophosphorus compounds

A number of organophosphorus compounds are still used for anthelmintic treatment and the majority of these were investigated originally as pesticides and only subsequently used as anthelmintics. Because of their potentially toxic action on the mammalian host they have to be used with care. The special formulation developed in the case of dichlorvos for treatment in the dog allows for slow release when given orally.

Mode of action

The main effect of all organophosphorus compounds on helminths is an inhibition of acetylcholinesterase production which leads to an interference in neuromuscular transmission. The symptoms of toxicity when it occurs in animals are usually frequent defecation and urination and muscular weakness. The likely toxic effect of any specific organophosphorus compound is related to the susceptibility of the mammalian acetylcholinesterase to the drug.

One organophosphorus anthelmintic, haloxon, appears to have a temporary effect on acetylcholine in the sheep so toxicity hazard is low at the therapeutic dose.

Dichlorvos

$$(CH_3O)_2\overset{\displaystyle O}{\overset{\|}{P}}—O—CH=CCl_2$$

Dichlorvos is incorporated into polyvinyl chloride resin pellets and the volatile drug is slowly released from the pellets as they pass down the intestines. This allows an effective level of drug to be released in dogs and horses and also ensures that there is time for detoxification to take place within the body without producing signs of toxicity.

Spectrum of activity

The compound is given to horses, dogs, cats and pigs. It is very effective in dogs and cats in the control of hookworms, ascarids and the whipworm. It is not active against larval stages of roundworms or tapeworm.

Dichlorvos is active in pigs against fourth-stage larvae and adults of *Ascaris suum*, the nodular worm *Oesophagostomum*, the whipworm *Trichuris suis* and the stomach worms *Hyostrongylus rubidus* and *Ascarops strongylina*.

In the horse it is active against the three large strongyles, ascarids and bot larvae which are found in the stomach. The drug is usually administered in the feed in pellet form for animal treatment.

Pharmacokinetics

Following oral administration of the pellets, the gradually released drug is absorbed and detoxified in the liver. The blood levels of organophosphorus compound remain below those likely to produce signs of inhibition of acetyl-cholinesterase in the treated animal. The drug is detoxified mainly to dichloroacetaldehyde but other metabolites probably also occur. The metabolites are excreted in the faeces and urine.

Toxicology

Toxic effects are infrequent when the drug is given at therapeutic levels. But it is important to avoid using the drug when other cholinesterase-inhibiting agents, such as pesticides, have been used. In addition, other agents such as tranquillizers and muscle relaxants which influence muscle action should also be avoided during treatment.

Haloxon

Haloxon was developed in the 1960s as an organophosphorus compound with a low toxic potential for sheep and cattle. Because the complex formed in sheep erythrocytes between acetylcholinesterase enzyme and haloxon can dissociate, the danger of toxicity is reduced.

Spectrum of activity

It is active against the majority of sheep and cattle nematodes but without the broad activity against larval stages shown by the benzimidazoles and ivermectin, so that its future use will depend on its comparative economic value.

Pharmacokinetics

As with other organophosphorus compounds, haloxon is absorbed quite readily and metabolized rapidly into non-toxic metabolites.

Toxicology

As with other organophosphorus compounds, haloxon should not be used on animals which have been or are under treatment with an organophosphorus pesticide.

Coumaphos and trichlorphon

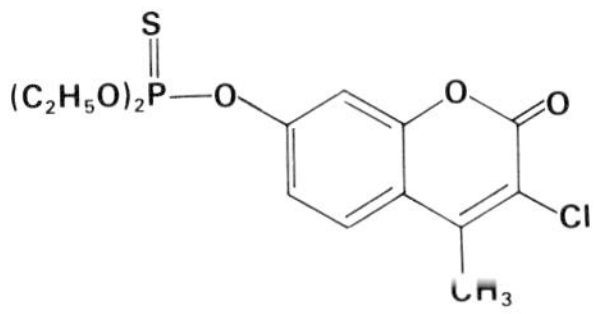

Coumaphos 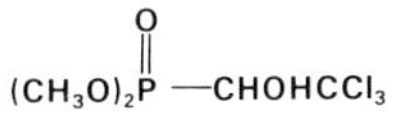   Trichlorphon

    Both these compounds were developed as pesticides and were tested as anthelmintics in the 1950s because of the relative inefficiency of phenothiazine as a broad-spectrum anthelmintic. They are now used as economical anthelmintics and trichlorphon has an advantage because of its activity against bots in the stomach of the horse. Coumaphos is used as a feed supplement for the treatment of beef and dairy cattle.

Anilides and substituted phenols

This group (Table 6.9) was developed as a result of the search for new chemicals which would have better and safer activity than carbon tetrachloride or hexachlorophane against the liver fluke in sheep and cattle. One member of the group, niclosamide, has no liver fluke activity but is active against tapeworms.

Table 6.9. Activities of anilides and phenol anthelmintics in sheep and cattle.

Site of activity	Worms	Spectrum				
		Oxy-clozanide	Rafox-anide	Niclos-amide	Diamphen-ethide	Nitroxy-nil
Stomach	*Haemonchus*					
	adult	1	4	–	–	3
	immature	–	3	–	–	–
Intestine	Tapeworm *Monezia*					
	adult	–	–	4	–	–
Liver	Liver fluke *Fasciola*					
	adult	4	4	–	3	4
	immature	2	4	–	4	2

Approximate efficiency ratings: $4 = 95–100\%$; $3 = 85–95\%$; $2 = 60–85\%$; $1 = 60\%$.

Oxyclozanide

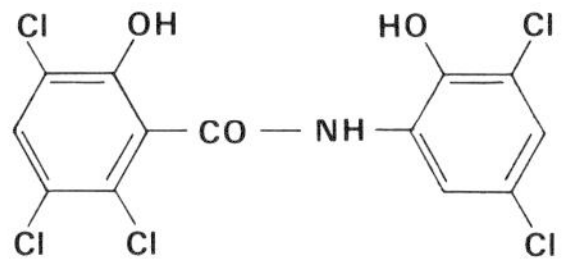

Cl OH   HO Cl
    — CO — NH —
Cl Cl   Cl

Oxyclozanide was the first of a group of new chemicals which were developed with specific action against the liver fluke. It was introduced in 1966 with specific action against adult flukes.

Mode of action

It acts against the parasite because it is an uncoupler of oxidative phosphorylation which leads to the death of adult flukes.

Pharmacokinetics

Oxyclozanide is absorbed readily and reaches high concentrations in the liver, kidneys and intestines. It is metabolized and excreted in the bile as an active glucuronide metabolite. It is relatively inactive against the larval stages of the fluke, possibly because of protein binding in the blood.

Toxicology

The recommended dose range for sheep and cattle is 10–15 mg/kg, which gives a safety margin of 6, as the maximum tolerated dose is 60 mg/kg. Safety is an important feature in liver fluke treatment, as many of the animals may have considerable liver damage at the time of treatment.

Rafoxanide

Toxicology

This drug is active against 99% of adult flukes and in the region of 86–99% of six-week-old flukes, so it has a reasonably broad spectrum against flukes.

Pharmacokinetics

Rafoxanide is usually given as an oral suspension. It is absorbed slowly and reaches a peak in the plasma at about 24 hours. It undergoes insignificant metabolism and has a half-life of 5–10 days in sheep.

As it appears in the milk, it must not be given to milking cows.

Rafoxanide has a safety margin of approximately 5 and the recommended dose by injection is 3 mg/kg and orally 7.5 mg/kg for sheep and cattle.

Because of the long half-life, there is a withholding time of 28 days following treatment.

Diamphenethide

Diamphenethide was the first chemical developed with specific activity against the very young immature flukes. This provided a drug which could be used when weather conditions favoured high infestations of young flukes early in the autumn. When such infestations are common they are often associated with bacterial infections of the liver due to clostridia. This can lead to a disease known as 'black disease' in sheep which can cause serious losses.

Pharmacokinetics

The chemical is given orally and rapidly absorbed and distributed throughout the body, with subsequent concentration in the liver. When it reaches the liver, diamphenethide is deacetylated by liver enzymes to an amine metabolite which is fatal to the young immature flukes. The metabolite is subsequently destroyed in the liver so that little of the drug activity reaches the bile ducts in which lie the mature flukes.

Toxicology

Although the dose of 100 mg/kg is relatively high, there is a good safety margin.

Nitroxynil

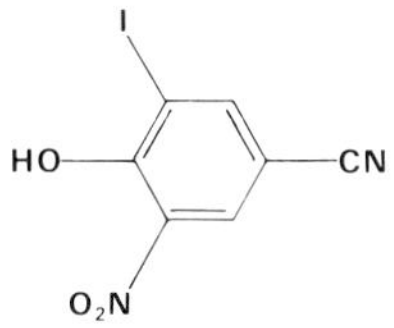

Nitroxynil was developed in the late 1960s as an injectable formula for liver fluke control. The drug is given by subcutaneous injection to cattle and sheep. Because of its slow elimination it cannot be given to lactating cows, and animals cannot be slaughtered for human consumption within 30 days of treatment.

Pharmacokinetics

The details of the pharmacology of nitroxynil have not been published but it has been suggested that it acts by uncoupling oxidative phosphorylation in the cells. It is very slowly eliminated from the body.

Nitroscanate

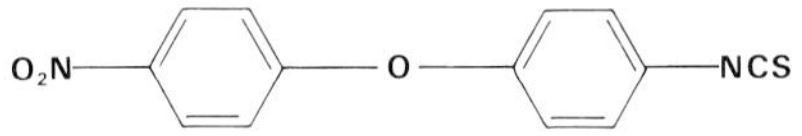

Nitroscanate is a broad-spectrum anthelmintic which is active against the major range of helminths which affect both cats and dogs.

The standard dosage is 50 mg/kg bodyweight, and the tablet is best given with a small amount of food. Vomiting may occasionally follow treatment.

Bunamidine

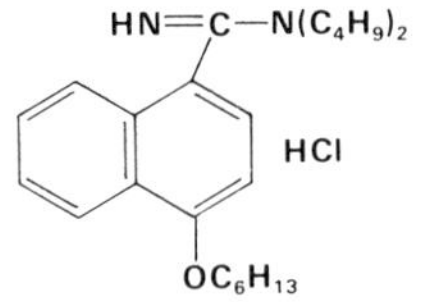

Bunamidine hydrochloride is active against the tapeworms of the dog.

Mode of action

The drug has the effect of disrupting the integument of the tapeworm, so that it is unable to take up glucose effectively. The tapeworm dies and is digested in the gut of the host.

Pharmacokinetics

The drug is given in the form of tablets designed to disintegrate only on reaching the stomach and it acts on the tapeworms in the small intestine. Ideally the drug should be slowly absorbed; too rapid absorption can produce toxic reactions. Bunamidine is metabolized in the liver.

Toxicology

Provided the tablet does not disintegrate until it reaches the stomach, no toxic reactions are found at normal dosing levels. The major toxic symptoms, vomiting and diarrhoea, seem to be associated with previous liver damage.

Other anthelmintics

Diethylcarbamazine

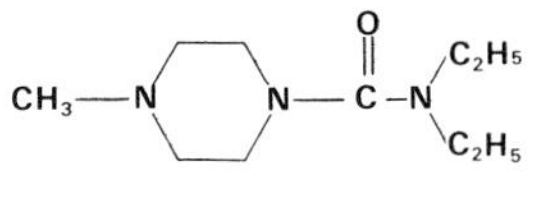

Diethylcarbamazine is a complex methylpiperazine derivative and is used in the form of the citrate salt. Its major use in therapy in the dog is in the prevention of heartworm disease. It is active against the third and fourth stage larvae.

The drug is given in the feed daily throughout the mosquito season and, in many cases, puppies may start on the drug as soon as they are weaned. Where adult dogs are already infected, preventive treatment for new infections must be preceded by treatment to eliminate adult filaria by dosing with thiacetarsamide or levamisole. Occasional dogs show an acute anaphylactic reaction if they are given diethylcarbamazine when they are already carrying an adult infection.

Mode of action

The drug appears to lead to paralysis of the nervous system of the larval stages of the heartworm *Dirofilaria immitis*.

Pharmacokinetics

It is rapidly absorbed from the gut and reaches a peak blood level within three hours. It is distributed throughout the body and is rapidly metabolized and excreted mainly through the urine.

Niclosamide

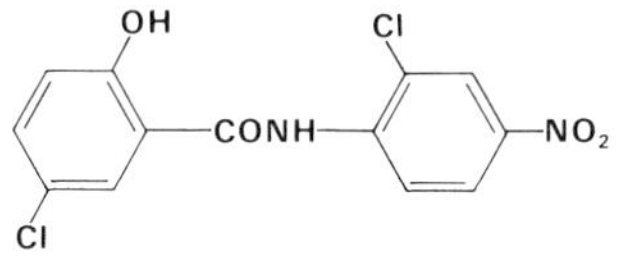

Niclosamide is active against the major tapeworms of domestic animals and when given in tablet form is poorly absorbed from the intestinal tract. Because it is poorly absorbed, the drug has a wide margin of safety.

Mode of action

The drug acts by inhibiting the absorption of glucose by the tapeworm. This is caused by a blocking of the Krebs cycle which leads to accumulation of lactic acid and the death of the tapeworm.

Piperazine salts

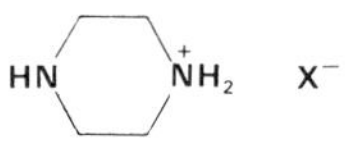

A range of piperazine salts such as the adipate, citrate and phosphate were developed in the 1950s as the first really safe anthelmintics for the control of roundworms in pigs, poultry, dogs, cats and horses. These salts all have wide margins of safety.

The drug is effective against the adult stages only, so that the treatment has to be repeated to ensure removal of all infection.

Mode of action

The piperazines act at the myoneural junction and have an anticholinergic effect. This produces a neuromuscular block and the result in the worm is a paralytic effect. The worms release their hold on the gut and are swept out.

Pharmacokinetics

The salts are readily absorbed from the gastro-intestinal tract and approximately 40% is excreted in the urine. The remainder is metabolized in the tissues.

Praziquantel

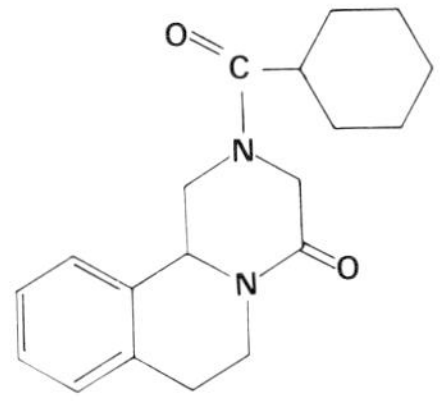

Praziquantel is active against the major tapeworms of the dog and cat and has the additional advantage of activity against many immature forms, including those of *Echinococcus granulosus*. It can be given orally as a tablet or by subcutaneous injection. The drug has a wide margin of safety.

Mode of action

Praziquantel acts by interfering with carbohydrate metabolism and can affect the tegument of the worm so that it becomes permeable, leading to excessive loss of glucose.

Pharmacokinetics

The drug is absorbed from the small intestine and reaches a peak blood level 30–60 minutes after administration. The action against tapeworm can occur both as a result of the presence of the drug in the intestines and as a result of re-excretion of the drug through the intestinal cells—in this way the attached head is affected. The drug is metabolized by the liver and excreted rapidly.

7. Pesticides

Introduction

A range of pesticides has been developed over the years to control the external parasites which are found on all animals whether they are kept extensively, such as sheep and cattle, or intensively like pigs and poultry, or as individuals in the case of the horse, dog and cat. The major problem areas where the control of parasites is vital are those where animals range over land which is favourable to the maintenance of parasite populations. These areas were recognized in the nineteenth century when the keeping of domestic cattle and sheep became of economic importance in the USA, South America, South Africa, Australia and New Zealand. It was found that ticks, for example, could transmit protozoal infections when attached, in addition to causing anaemia because of blood loss. In Australia the blowfly, known in the UK as the maggot fly, caused death in sheep which were subject to larval attack when they were already in poor condition as a result of intercurrent infections due to worm infestations, foot rot or pregnancy toxaemia, an acute disease of late pregnancy.

Table 7.1.   Common pests of domestic animals.

Species	Parasites			
Cattle	hornfly and other biting flies warble fly screwworm fly	lice	ticks	mites
Sheep	blowfly headfly nasal bot fly keds	lice	ticks	mites
Pigs	biting flies	lice	ticks	mites
Horses	biting flies bot fly	lice	ticks	mites
Poultry		lice	ticks	mites	fleas
Dogs and cats		lice	ticks	mites	fleas

The regular use of pesticides was, therefore, recognized as an essential part of the maintenance of large herds of cattle or flocks of sheep. At the same time the control of the infestations of lice and fleas on domestic animals became common.

In the USA it is reckoned that more than 500 million dollars are lost annually because of animal parasite infestations and worldwide this may amount to 7 billion dollars when the losses associated with the extensive farming practised in South America, Australia, New Zealand and South Africa are considered.

All external parasites pass through a number of stages in their life cycle and can be classified as Arachnida or Insecta. The Arachnida include ticks and mites and each parasite in its development passes through egg, larval, nymphal and adult stages. The Insecta, which includes flies, lice and fleas, pass through egg, larval, pupal and adult stages. It is only by an understanding of the significance of each stage that it is possible to develop a pesticide programme for their control.

Arachnida

Ticks

The ticks can be attacked practically with a pesticide only when they are on the host, and control is influenced by the fact that the different species of ticks may live on only one host for their whole lives, or on two or three different hosts. Spraying of the environment in addition to the treatment of animals for tick control is impracticable with sheep and cattle because of the vast area grazed by the animals and because of possible hazard to the environment posed by the presence of an insecticide on the ground.

The adult female one-host ticks such as *Boophilus* (Figures 7.1 and 7.4), after engorging on cattle, drop off and lay their eggs on the ground. The subsequent stages (larva, nymph and adult, male and female) all live on one animal and must attach to the skin to engorge blood. The larval and nymphal stages do not fall to the ground after engorgement but remain attached to the host. Dipping is usually practised at intervals of 21 days as this period covers the 20-day life cycle when the parasites are on the host.

In two-host ticks such as *Rhipicephalus* (Figure 7.5) and *Hyalomma* (Figure 7.2), the engorged female drops to the ground and lays it eggs. After hatching from the eggs, the larva attaches to the host, feeds and then moults to a nymph while still on the host. The nymph emerges and feeds on the same host, then drops to the ground and the next moult to the adult stage takes place off the host. The newly emerged adult has then to attach to a new host before completing its life cycle. Control of the two-host tick requires dipping at seven-day intervals if all stages of the tick on the animal at the time are to be killed.

Three-host ticks such as *Amblyomma* (Figure 7.3) and *Ixodes*, have to find

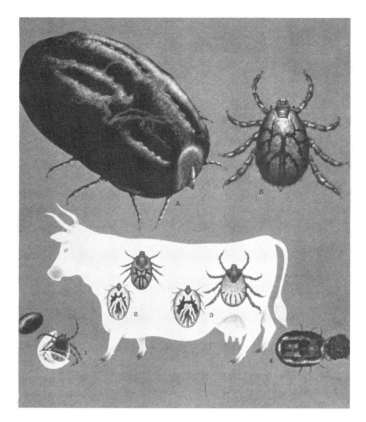

Figure 7.1. Life cycle of one-host cattle tick *Boophilus* spp. A: The engorged female. B: The male.

1. Larvae hatch from the eggs. Seven to ten days later the larvae climb the vegetation and seek a host.

2. They attach to their host and engorge on its blood within three to five days. They then pass into a moult. Two days later nymphs emerge from the moult and also take a blood meal lasting five to six days.

3. The engorged nymphs pass into a two-day moult from which adult males and females emerge. Fertilization takes place. The female then feeds for a period of five to seven days and during the last 24 hours completes engorgement with a large blood feed.

4. The engorged female drops to the ground 20 or more days after attaching as a larva and seeks a suitable place to lay her eggs. 2000 eggs are laid in a humid niche on the ground.

new hosts at the larval, nymphal and adult stages. Complete control can be achieved only by dipping every 5–7 days.

Mites

A range of mites attack farm and domestic animals (Figure 7.6) but, unlike the two- and three-host ticks, mites once on the host complete their life cycle

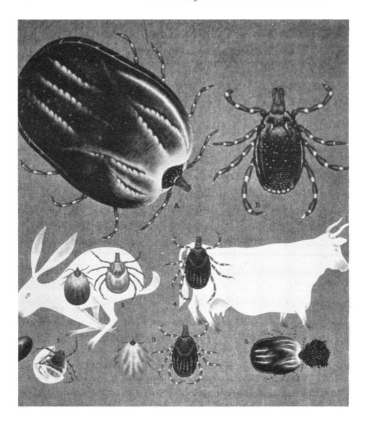

Figure 7.2.   Life cycle of two-host cattle tick *Hyalomma* spp.
A: The engorged female. B: The male.
1. Larvae hatch from eggs which are laid on the ground and several days later they seek a host, often a small animal such as a hare, although birds and mammals of all sizes may be hosts to immature *Hyalomma*.
2. The larvae attach to their host and engorg on its blood before moulting to nymphs. The nymphs in turn take a blood meal from the host.
3. The engorged nymphs drop to the ground to moult. Males and females emerge from this moult and find a large animal host.
4. They attach, often in the anal or vulval regions. Fertilization takes place on the host and the female then completes a large blood meal.
5. The engorged female drops to the ground five to seven days after attaching and lays c.10 000 eggs in a suitable place. *Hyalomma* are tolerant of a wider range of conditions, particularly drought, than many hard ticks. They may also change the feeding habits of their life cycle to avoid unfavourable conditions.

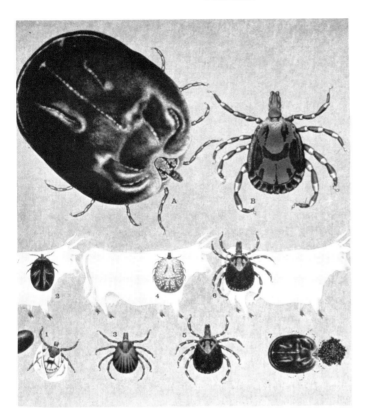

Figure 7.3.   Life cycle of three-host cattle tick *Amblyomma* spp. A: The engorged female. B: The male.

1. Larvae hatch from eggs that are laid on the ground and several days later climb the vegetation to seek a host.

2. The larvae attach to a host, usually on the hairy parts of the head or body and engorge with blood.

3. The engorged larvae drop to the ground to moult. Nymphs emerge from this moult.

4. The nymphs attach to another host on similar sites and engorge with blood.

5. The engorged nymphs drop to the ground to moult. The ornate males and females emerge from this moult.

6. They find a third host and attach, often in the groins, on the scrotum or udder, anus, vulva or escutcheon. Fertilization takes place on the host after which the female engorges with blood.

7. The engorged female drops to the ground seven to ten days after attaching and lays eggs in a sheltered humid place on the ground. One engorged female of the large African species such as *A variegatum* may lay 20 000 eggs.

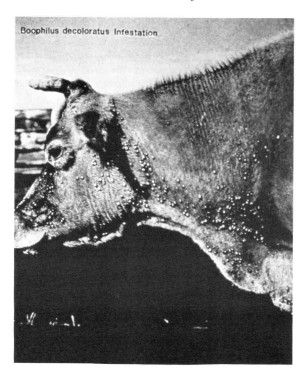

Figure 7.4.   Infestation of *Boophilus decoloratus* one-host tick—neck of cattle.

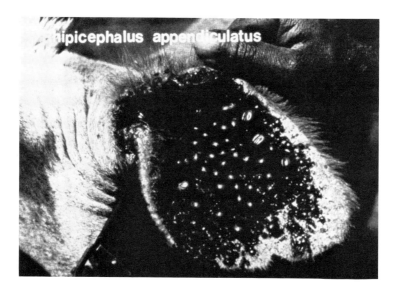

Figure 7.5 (*a*) Infestation of *Rhipicephalus appendiculatus* a three-host tick—in the ear of cattle.

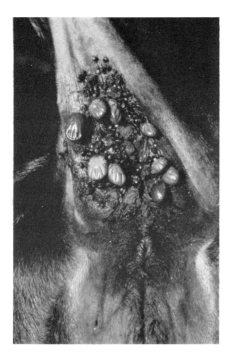

Figure 7.5 (*b*) Infestation of *Rhipicephalus evertsi* under cattle tail.

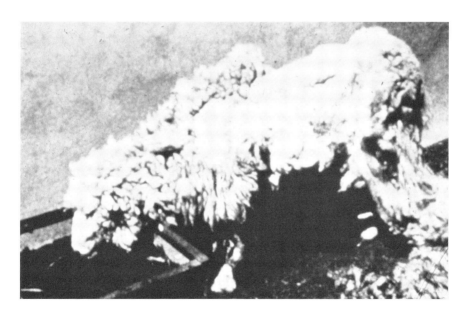

Figure 7.6. Sheep scab mite infestation.

on the one animal. So a single dipping with an insecticide which persists in the wool is usually an effective means of control. For sheep, the dip should be applied shortly after shearing so that the maximum penetration is obtained. Additional dipping in both sheep and cattle may be necessary where heavy infestations exist, or where complete mustering of sheep at dipping time cannot be guaranteed.

Insecta

The insects pass through egg, larval and an inactive pupal stage before becoming adults. In the case of flies which attack animals (Figures 7.7–7.9), damage to the host can occur in one of two ways, either during the larval stage when the parasite feeds on the tissues of the host, for example blowfly or nasal bot fly, or in the case of the hornfly, stable fly, face fly and head fly, by irritation of the host as the adult punctures the skin in the search for flood. Unlike the other insects, the ked (Figure 7.10), which is found on sheep, spends its whole life on its host because it has lost its wings.

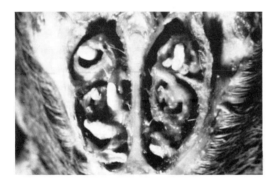

Figure 7.7.   Nasal bot fly larvae—sheep.

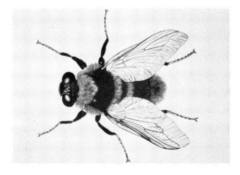

Figure 7.8.   Cattle—warble fly (*Hypoderma bovis*).

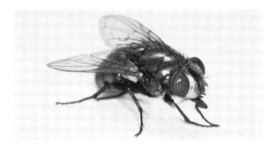

Figure 7.9 (*a*) *Lucilia sericata*—sheep blow fly.

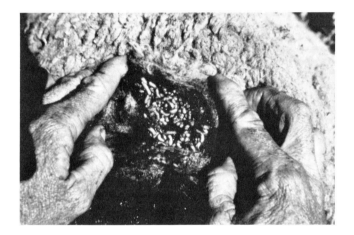

Figure 7.9 (*b*) Blow fly strike on sheep.

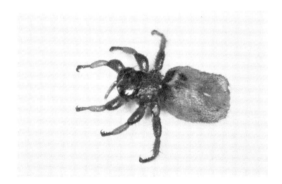

Figure 7.10.   Sheep ked.

Control

Where the control of the larval stage of a fly is the problem the host (usually a sheep) is dipped or sprayed with an insecticide which will persist in the fleece and kill the larvae which have hatched from the eggs in the fleece, before they can penetrate the skin. In the case of biting fly attacks, regular spraying of cattle and horses during the active summer period is used to deter the fly, or back rubbers impregnated with insecticide are placed at strategic sites on a property, or impregnated ear tags are placed in the ears.

Both lice (Figure 7.11) and keds, which live entirely on the host, can be controlled by spraying, showering or dipping shortly after shearing. Fleas, which develop off the host during the egg, larval and nymphal stages and appear on the host only as adults, can be controlled by dusting and spraying likely egg-laying sites so that the larval stages are killed when on the move within the treat area, and by treating the host using dusts, dips or insecticidal collars.

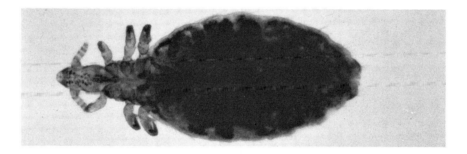

Figure 7.11 (*a*) Sucking louse of sheep (*Linognathus ovillus*).

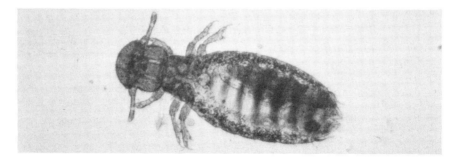

Figure 7.11 (*b*) Biting louse of sheep (*Damalinia ovis*).

Damage to the host

The amount of damage caused to the host by parasites is dependent on the activity of the various stages of the parasite. For example, larval stages which migrate through the tissues of the host can cause considerable damage for a long period. Mange mites cause superficial damage by burrowing into the skin layer, but this may lead to economic loss as a result of irritation which forces the host to respond by continual itching and scratching. In sheep this may cause the wool to fall out.

Whatever the sequence of events, all parasites, when present in significant numbers, can do considerable damage to an animal. Economically, the cattle tick probably causes more damage to the farming industry than any other single parasite. It is ubiquitous throughout the semi-tropical and tropical parts of the world and, in drought periods, can cause serious emaciation and death to many thousand cattle, because in addition to sucking blood, the tick transmits a number of protozoal infections via the blood stream.

Use of pesticides

The early chemicals (such as sulphur, arsenic, derris and nicotine) used for the control of parasites were difficult to deal with in the field, as high concentrations of active principle were needed in dip baths and the chemicals could produce toxic effects even when used at the recommended concentration. It was therefore a major advance in animal parasite control when highly specific insecticides, such as DDT and benzene hexachloride were introduced for use in animals. In addition to being active against the major parasites they had a residual effect on the wool and hair which was sufficient to kill larval stages which attached to an animal following dipping or which hatched from an egg shortly after treatment commenced.

It is possible to define an ideal insecticide based on experience acquired during the last 30 years of usage.
(1) It should destroy all stages of a parasite on the animal.
(2) Its action should be rapid.
(3) It should be safe in use and leave no toxic residues.
(4) It should be stable in dip tanks and spraying machines and remain active under the extremes of temperature in tropical conditions.
(5) It should not pose an environmental hazard.

Pesticidal formulations and methods of application

The formulation of pesticides is a very specialized art as the suspensions or emulsions which are required for use in dip tanks or sprays have to withstand

Table 7.2.   Methods of application of peticides. See also Figures 7.12–7.16.

	Method of application	Type of applicators
Cattle	Dips	Large tanks—8000–20 000 litres
	Sprays	Races and hand applied sprayers
	Dusters	Power dusters similar to those used in plant treatments
	Back rubbers	The pesticide is formulated in oil and applied by the cattle themselves as they rub against the impregnated sacking
	Pour-on preparations for systemic effect	The application is poured onto the back of the animal
	Ear tag	Polyvinyl insecticide impregnated tag fixed in the ear
Sheep	Dips	Large and small tanks
	Showers	Overhead rotating power sprays
	Sprays	High- and low-pressure sprays
	Jetting	High-power jet of suspension applied to selected areas—tail and back of sheep
	Dusting	Power dusters
Pigs	Sprays	Low-pressure sprays
	Pour-on preparations	Syringe or pressure container
	Powders	In feed
Horses	Dips	Similar to cattle
	Sprays	Hand held, or tunnel spray races
	Pour-on or sponge-on preparations for systemic effect	The pesticide is sponged onto the back and sides
Dogs and cats	Shampoos	Suspendable powders, emulsions
	Washes	Suspendable powders, emulsions
	Dusts	Hand dusters
	Flee and tick collars	

stresses which are not encountered in other areas of veterinary medicine. The final diluted formulation used in a dip tank or spray race must, in spite of being contaminated with soil and faeces throughout the dipping or spraying process, remain stable in a dip bath or tank for many months. During this time it will often be further diluted by rainwater. It will also be expected to pass through high-pressure nozzles and be continually agitated.

The methods of application of pesticides for animal use have evolved over the years to suit both new management systems and the individual requirements of dog and cat owners. Some of the methods of application are mentioned in Table 7.2.

Resistance to pesticides

Many of the newer pesticides have been developed as a response to the appearance of insect resistance following the use of earlier insecticides on animal or cereal pests. Resistance is recognized as an inevitable hazard of

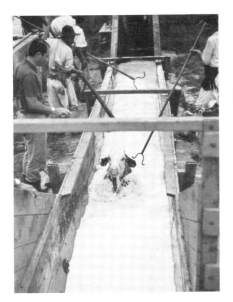

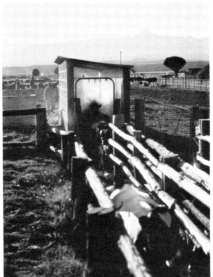

Figure 7.12.   Cattle dipping.   Figure 7.13.   Cattle spraying.

the wide use of an insecticide. Brown and Pal (1971) said that "resistance in the field is a measurable quantity, and results from a change in the genotype composition of an insect population, which follows on the selection pressure exerted by insecticides. When a significant amount of resistance is recognized in an insect population then it is essential to change to a different compound. Although there will be grades of resistance, there is an inherent danger in the continual use of an insecticide in a population which it is hoped to control."

Resistance, when it occurs, is present in both adult and larval stages and the resistance is transmitted genetically. The speed of its establishment will depend on whether the genes are dominant or recessive. In some cases the resistance can be bred out in six generations by rearing the insect in the absence of the compound. In general, resistant strains of parasites form a minority of the original population. In the testing of insecticides it is common practice now to study the effect of a new insecticide on the physiological functions of individual species of parasites so that the possibility of resistance developing can be recognized in advance.

In practice, therefore, it is still essential that the search for new insecticides be maintained if a continuing programme of parasite control is to be achieved. Should resistance occur with an established insecticide it is usual to mix two insecticides, sometimes even two organophosphorus compounds to achieve an improved effect. The original resistance may have occurred when one or other insecticide has been used on its own.

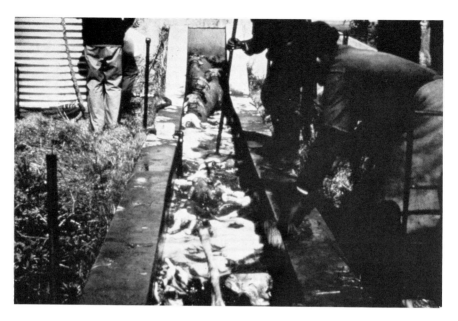

Figure 7.14.   Sheep dipping.

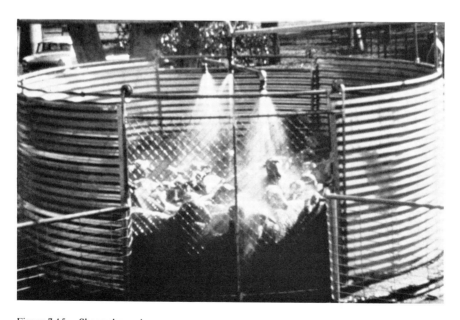

Figure 7.15.   Sheep showering.

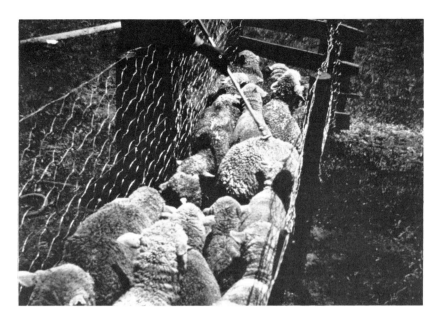

Figure 7.16.   Sheep jetting.

Mode of action of pesticides used in animal treatment

Because many of the pesticides used for animal treatment were developed for the control of both plant and animal parasites, very detailed studies have been made of the mode of action of each pesticide or pesticide group on the individual parasites. Study of the mechanism of insecticide action has two important functions. Firstly, it establishes the pathway by which a toxic effect is achieved in the insect. Secondly, should resistance develop, it gives a guide as to which systems have to be investigated to establish how an insect is able to prevent a toxic effect when exposed to a normally active dose of insecticide.

The action of insecticides is similar in both arachnids and insects provided that the parasite to be treated is sensitive to the insecticide which is to be used. The specific action can be described under a number of headings and is mainly associated with an interference with the normal transmission of nerve impulses (Corbett *et al.* 1983).

The nerve cell (Figure 7.17) conducts the impulses by which the nervous system functions. Each nerve cell has a nucleus surrounded by cytoplasm, and this constitutes the cell body. From the cell body project thread-like processes which carry the impulses from place to place. Each process consists of a single axon and the transfer to another nerve cell of the impulse which travels on the axon takes place at the synapse. Here a chemical substance

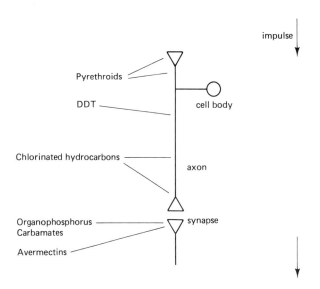

Figure 7.17.   Schematic plan of a nerve cell (neurone).

called a neurotransmitter is released by the active cell to cross the gap (the synapse) to the next cell and activate it in turn. One important neurotransmitter is acetylcholine. When this has done its job, it is destroyed by the enzyme acetylcholinesterase—any substance that interferes with this enzyme will clearly disrupt the overall functioning of the nervous system.

Pesticides can act on different parts of the nerve transmission process. The pyrethroids interfere with transmission along the axon, whereas benzene hexachloride (BHC) causes release of excess acetylcholine at the end of the axon. Organophosphorus compounds, carbamates and avermectins interfere with the transmission of nerve impulses at the synapses. The five main types of action are as follows.

1. Interference with axonal transmission

Effect of pyrethroids

The pyrethroids interfere with an insect's normal nervous activity and this is seen when treated insects show greatly increased activity followed by unco-ordinated action and eventually paralysis. This is caused by disruption of axonal conduction of impulses. The disruption is related to the movement of sodium and potassium ions leading to a prolongation of the inward sodium current which has a significant effect on the electric potential of the nerve cell.

The delayed closing of the sodium channels affects the neurones, and probably acts directly on muscle contraction. The increased nervous and muscular activity is followed by other events in the body, such as dehydration, which will lead to the death of the insect.

Effect of DDT

DDT, like the pyrethroids, acts on the neurones by prolonging the inward sodium current and preventing the potassium/sodium exchange which is necessary to maintain normal neurone action. Instead of the normal flow of nerve impulses, there is high repetitive activity which leads to excitability and eventual exhaustion of the treated insect. It is known too that DDT causes a release of hormones which can affect the metabolism of the insect. Because of the very similar biochemical action of pyrethroids and DDT, insects with a resistance factor due to an alteration at the site of action of DDT are also resistant to pyrethroids.

2. Excessive release of acetylcholine

The neurotoxicity of Gamma BHC, which is shown by violent quivering of the insect body followed by convulsions and paralysis, is due to excessive release of acetylcholine leading to hyperactivity at cholinergic synapses.

3. Stimulation of motor output from insect ganglia

Amitraz stimulates the motor output from insect ganglia and this gives rise to the production of dimethylformamidine. This chemical produces a toxic effect which increases activity and causes ticks to detach from treated hosts, thus achieving the desired parasite clearance from the animal.

4. Interference with synapses at which GABA (γ-amino butyric acid) is the transmitter

GABA acts as an inhibitory transmitter and tends to reduce excitability in the post-synapse cells. The insecticidal and anthelmintic effect of the avermectins is seen as a paralysis of the parasites due to the blocking of GABA transmissions.

5. Inhibition of acetylcholinesterase

Organophosphorus and carbamate compounds react with acetyl-cholinesterase by forming a reversibe complex with the enzyme. Elimination of the leaving groups follows, to give a derivative of the enzyme in which serine is phosphorylated. A carbamate likewise leads to a carbamylated enzyme. The enzyme derivatives are unable to carry out the essential hydrolysis of acetylcholine which therefore accumulates.

Despite the many studies on both organophosphorus and carbamate actions, it is difficult to establish the precise chain of events between inhibition of the enzyme and insect death. The excess of acetylcholine can have widespread effects on the insect, particularly due to uncontrolled hormone release. This can lead to degeneration of vital tissues and loss of water leading to dehydration.

Arsenicals

Dips containing arsenic were the first to be widely used throughout the world for the control of the parasites of both sheep and cattle. Arsenic trioxide (As_2O_3) was inexpensive and readily soluble in water, and there was a simple test which could be used at the time of dipping to establish the concentration present in the dip fluid. A final concentration of 0·32% active ingredient was found to be effective and relatively safe.

Arsenic, although active against ticks following dipping, would protect against re-infestation only for 10–12 hours after treatment. It had the disadvantage that arsenic as a concentrate was highly poisonous and dangerous to handle and could, if used at over-strength, cause severe burning of the skin in cattle and death by absorption in sheep which had been dipped in cold, wet weather which did not allow rapid drying of the fleece. In the 1950s, many cases of tick resistance to arsenic were being encountered in Australia, USA and South Africa so that the more effective modern insecticides have steadily replaced arsenic.

Chlorinated hydrocarbons

Gamma BHC   DDT

The group of chlorinated hydrocarbons was the first of the highly specific pesticides to become available generally in the 1950s for animal treatment. The best known, DDT, had established its reputation during the war when its use protected the allied troops from infestation of lice (the carrier of the typhus organism) in Naples during the outbreak of typhus which killed many civilians.

The major organochlorines now used for animal treatment are gamma BHC (lindane) and campheclor (toxaphene). Aldrin and dieldrin are also highly effective organochlorines, particularly in the control of sheep parasites, because they persist in the fleece for many months. However, their use was eventually banned in all the major animal-producing countries because residual deposits of chemical were found in body tissues and in the milk of animals treated in a dip. In addition, by 1959 many parasites, particularly the sheep blowfly and some ticks, were showing resistance to both insecticides. Of the organochlorines originally developed and for-mulated for animal use, only two are now still in general use—lindane and toxaphene.

Gamma benzene hexachloride (lindane)

Gamma benzene hexachloride is the gamma isomer of 1,2,3,4,5,6-hexachloro-chlorocyclohexane and is used for animal treatment as a spray, dip and dust. As a spray and dip it is applied at a concentration of 0·03 to 0·05% in water. It is formulated either as a wettable powder which will mix readily with water and will remain suspended in a dip for sufficient time for the particles to attach to the fleece or skin, or as a liquid concentrate which mixes with water.

It is important that dip suspensions containing lindane are regularly renewed during the dipping process as the dip particles are removed in the fleece and fouling of the wash can cause degradation of the active material. In addition, the dip must contain a bacteriostat to prevent infection in sheep with the organism *Erysipelothrix rhusiopathiae*. This organism is ubiquitous in nature and can cause skin infection on the legs of sheep the skin of which has been broken during dipping.

Gamma benzene hexachloride is still used as a general spray for the control of parasites on cattle, pigs and dogs and as a dip for the control of the sheep scab mite. It has proved to be very safe in use and the only toxic hazard occurs in very young animals such as puppies and kittens.

Toxaphene (chlorinated camphene, $C_{10}H_{10}Cl_8$)

Toxaphene is used as a spray, dip, back rubber or dust and is active against the major animal parasites found in the USA, South America, Africa and Australia.

Spray and dip formulations are used at a concentration of 0·3 to 0·5%. The chemical, which is a sticky resinous material, is stable in dip and spray washes and adheres well to the coat and skin, so that a good residual effect is obtained. Sufficient chemical may be retained on the skin during dipping to kill parasites which attach four days after treatment.

Toxaphene is also used as a back rubber for the control of hornfly in the USA. The toxaphene is added to a reservoir container, and is absorbed by a cloth wick which supplies insecticide to the back rubber.

Although strains of ticks resistant to toxaphene have been found, this chemical is still used in the USA, South America, Africa and Australia.

Because of resistance, both toxaphene and lindane are frequently combined with organophosphorus compounds in dip tanks.

Toxaphene is more toxic than gamma benzene hexachloride, so has to be used with care and is not advised for young animals. It must not be used on dairy cattle or poultry. Animals should not be treated within 60 days of slaughter.

Organophosphorus compounds

Because the majority of the chlorinated hydrocarbons were withdrawn from general use in the mid 1950s, a gap was created in the whole field of parasite control. Fortunately the organophosphorus range of pesticides became available, and of the many thousands tested, 20 or more are in general use for animal treatment (Table 7.3). They are used on their own or in combination.

Although all organophosphorus compounds are potentially toxic to mammals, including man, in practice the pesticides used for animals have proved to be remarkably safe in use provided they are handled with care and used at the proper concentration. When an organophosphorus compound enters the body of an animal, the compound is metabolized and excreted in the urine. In the mammal unlike the insect, an enzyme is secreted when organophosphorus compound activity is recognized, and the active material is destroyed by hydrolysis and oxidation.

Should a toxic reaction occur in an animal under treatment the action can be reversed by the use of atropine and 2-pyridine aldoxime methiodide (2-PAM). As a precaution, very young animals and animals in poor condition or under stress, for example, in drought conditions, should be treated with care. The pesticide can be applied selectively to obviously infested areas.

Carbamates

A number of carbamates are used for animal treatment both on farm animals and dogs and cats—these include carbaryl (1-naphthyl *N*-methyl carbamate), isoprocarb (2-isopropylphenyl methyl carbamate) and propoxur (*O*-isopropoxyphenyl methyl carbamate). They are used on their own or more frequently in combination with pyrethrins, particularly in dog collars, when a quick knock-down is required.

Carbaryl   Isoprocarb   Propoxur

Table 7.3. Organophosphorus compounds in common use on farm animals.

Generic name	Spray	Dip	Pour-on	Dust	Back rubber	Mineral mix or feed	Ear tags
						Method of common use	
Chlorfenvinphos	×	×	−	−	−	−	
Chlorpyrifos	×	×	×	−	−	−	×
Coumaphos	×	×	×	×	×	−	
Crotoxyphos	×	−	−	×	×	−	
Crufomate	×	×	×	−	−	−	
Diazinon	×	×	−	−	−	−	
Dichlorvos	×	−	−	−	×	−	
Dichlorfenthion	×	×	−	−	−	×	
Dimethoate	×	×	×	×	×	×	
Diathion	×	×	−	−	×	−	
Ethion	×	×	−	−	−	−	
Famphur	−	−	×	×	−	−	
Fenchlorphos	−	−	×	×	−	−	
Fenthion	−	−	×	−	−	−	
Malathion	×	×	−	×	×	−	
Phosmet	×	×	×	−	−	−	
Ronnel	×	−	×	−	×	×	
Stirofos	×	−	−	×	×	×	
Trichlorfon	×	−	×	−	−	×	
Tetrachlorvinphos						×	

Mode of action

Kuhr and Dorough (1976) have discussed the action of carbamates as compared with organophosphorus compound in detail. The carbamates react with acetylcholinesterase, forming a carbamylated enzyme. The enzyme is unable to deal efficiently with the burst of acetylcholine liberated within the insect, so that proper nerve function is disrupted. In the case of carbamates, spontaneous reactivation of inhibited acetylcholinesterase can be measured in minutes, whereas the inhibition may last for hours in the case of organo-phosphorus compounds.

Carbamates are broken down in the body by blood esterases when they are circulating in the blood, and liver microsomal enzymes also break down the compounds very rapidly. Should signs of toxicity occur, the affected animal responds well to treatment with atropine.

Amitraz

Amitraz is a triazapentadiene and is used particularly for the treatment of tick-infested cattle.

Amitraz [1,5-di-(2,4-dimethylphenyl)-3-methyl-1,3,5-triazapenta-1,4-diene]

It is stable in dip baths provided the pH is kept high. Amitraz is particularly useful against the major ticks, and has proved safe in use in the field.

Chlormethiuron and chlordimeform

To counter resistance problems, a number of chemicals which have marked insecticidal activity have been added to organophosphorus dip bath formulations with success. They include chlormethiuron and chlordimeform.

Chlormethiuron   Chlordimeform

Chlormethiuron and chlordimeform appear to act by uncoupling oxidative phosphorylation or by inhibiting monoamine oxidase or by interfering with the action of octopamine, the neurophysiological role of which is being generally recognized.

Pyrethroids

This series includes the natural pyrethrins which are obtained from pyrethrum flowers and the new synthetic pyrethroids.

Pyrethrum is the extract of the active pyrethrins from the pyrethrum flower. Because of its relatively poor kill of parasites following a knock-down effect, it is usually combined with piperonyl butoxide, a synergist which ensures kill as well as knock-down effect. Pyrethrum itself always has a very short-term activity because of its instability in light.

The new synthetic pyrethroids are photostable and have considerable persistence so that they are largely replacing pyrethrum (Table 7.4).

Mode of action

The early synthetic pyrethrin, allethrin, when applied to the giant axons in the nerve cord of the cockroach, leads to an increase in the negative after-

Table 7.4. Structures of pyrethroids used for animal treatment.

Cypermethrin	$Cl_2C{=}CH$—[cyclopropane, Me, Me]—COOCH(CN)—[phenyl]—O—[phenyl]
Deltamethrin	$Br_2C{=}CH$—[cyclopropane, Me, Me]—COOCH(CN)—[phenyl]—O—[phenyl]
Permethrin	$Cl_2C{=}CH$—[cyclopropane, Me, Me]—$COOCH_2$—[phenyl]—O—[phenyl]
Fenvalerate	Cl—[phenyl]—$CHCOOCH$ with $CH(CH_3)_2$ and CN—[phenyl]—O—[phenyl]

potential and eventually blocks conduction. This appears to be due to blocking of some of the sodium, leading to continuous slow polarization and eventually the blocking of nervous conduction.

In general, the pyrethroids delay the closing of the sodium channels and this leads to the membrane potential difference becoming more positive so that the negative after-potential is increased. In addition, some pyrethroids may act directly on muscle and block normally stimulated neural/muscle action. The effect of the abnormal nervous activity is to induce a number of secondary effects and among these is dehydration due to water loss.

The action of the pyrethroids bears a similarity to that of DDT and it has been found that many insects which show resistance to DDT are also resistant to pyrethroids. Because of this, pyrethroid resistance has been encountered in ticks in Australia and it is recommended where this occurs that the pyrethroids be combined with a suitable organophosphorus compound to overcome the immediate problem. Alternatively, the pyrethroids can be used at a higher strength.

Uses of pyrethroids

Permethrin, fenvalerate and cypermethrin are used as sprays for tick control and fenvalerate is used for incorporation in ear tags for the control of the *Amblyomma* tick.

Cypermethrin, deltamethrin and permethrin are active against lice and keds.

Permethrin is used particularly for the control of biting flies on cattle and sheep.

Avermectins

The avermectins have been discussed in Chapter 6 under anthelmintics, so that in this section, mention will be made only of the activity of ivermectin against external parasites, which has been well reviewed by Campbell *et al.* (1983). The main activities are listed in Table 7.5. Although activity against all the parasites listed has been described, work is still in progress to determine the best way in which ivermectin can be formulated to provide a sustained effect against such parasites as ticks and blowfly.

Table 7.5.   Major parasites which can be treated with ivermectin.

Host	Parasites				
Cattle	mites	ticks	flies	lice	
Sheep	mites		sheep blowfly		keds
Pigs	mites			lice	
Dogs	mites				

At present, ivermectin is formulated mainly as a viscous solution containing 1% w/v ivermectin for subcutaneous injection in cattle, sheep, horses and pigs. In this form it is recommended for the treatment of internal parasites and such external parasites as warble fly larvae, lice, mites and ticks in cattle, and lice and mites in sheep.

For horses a 2% w/v solution is available for intramuscular injection, and also a 1·87% paste for oral dosing.

8. Coccidiostats and other antiprotozoal drugs

Coccidia

Coccidia are intracellular protozoal parasites most frequently found in the intestinal epithelial cells of vertebrates, but also found in the liver in some animals such as the rabbit. They are transmitted by faecal infection. Under natural conditions, infection in poultry is spread during the early days in the life of the chick when there is regular contact between the hen and her brood, and the infection is spread by faecal contamination of the ground by the carrier mother hen. The infective potential of coccidia in poultry is most important when the chicks are brought together in large numbers in intensive housing during broiler rearing. Coccidiosis is now so important in poultry production that commercial chicken feeds throughout the world contain anticoccidial agents as a normal constituent.

Nine species of coccidia have been identified in chickens and the main ones listed below all belong to the genus *Eimeria*.

E. acervulina	*E. mivati*
E. brunetti	*E. necatrix*
E. hagoni	*E. praecox*
E. maxima	*E. tenella*

As most coccidia types are found in the environment of any broiler unit, a new chemical developed for use as a coccidiostat must have proven activity against all the coccidia mentioned.

Coccidia pass through three phases in their development: *sporogony*, *schizogony* and *gametogony* (Figure 8.1). Sporogony occurs outside the host on the ground and consists of the forming of eight sporozoites in a sporulated oocyst. The oocyst is ingested by the host (the chick) and the eight sporozoites emerge from the oocyst in the digestive tract and then invade the epithelial cells of the intestine.

Each sporozoite in the cell undergoes what is called *schizogony* (reproduction by multiple asexual fission) and within two days becomes a *schizont* which then reproduces asexually by multiple fission and produces a number of *merozoites*. The merozoites escape from the cell and invade new cells

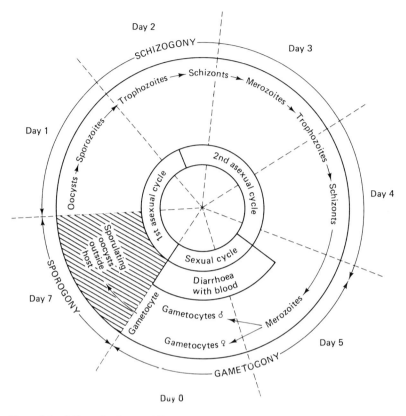

Figure 8.1.   Life cycle of a coccidium.

where they go through several stages of schizogony (separation of cells) over the next three days. This stage is followed by *gametogony* (production of a reproductive germ cell) which is the start of the sexual cycle of development. Two sexually different cells, macrogamonts and microgamonts, are formed. The macrogamont produces a single macrogamete (female) and the microgamont produces a number of microgametocytes (males). The microgametocytes fertilize the macrogametes and a zygote (the fertilized ovum before it undergoes cleavage) is produced which forms an oocyst wall and becomes an oocyst. This is then released into the lumen of the intestine and is discharged in the faeces to restart the life cycle.

The damage to the intestinal cell wall which is the cause of the acute disease of coccidiosis occurs between the fifth and sixth day after infection, when the merozoites start to invade cells and go through the schizogony which leads to gametogony.

Control of coccidiosis by chemotherapy

Once drugs became available which were likely to be effective in the treatment and control of coccidiosis, systems of testing these drugs were developed which demonstrated their efficacy both in artificial infections and under practical farm conditions. It soon became clear as more active drugs were found that treatment after infection had been recognized was not sufficiently effective in large poultry units, so research was concentrated on demonstrating systems of therapy which would prevent clinical disease ever appearing in a poultry unit.

As the aim in a broiler unit is to achieve permanent prevention of disease, it is usual to incorporate a coccidiostat in the feed throughout the entire 8–9 week growing period of the broiler. It is important, therefore, to use coccidiostats which are rapidly eliminated from the body so that any chemical residue at the time of slaughter is minimal.

Where poultry are being kept for longer periods, for example as egg layers or replacement stock, it is important to control infection without at the same time interfering with the development of natural immunity. Under these circumstances complete prevention of disease is not always practised. This can be achieved in three ways:

(1) A preventive dose of a coccidiostat at a level slightly lower than the dose given to a broiler is given for periods of between 6 and 22 weeks. In this way disease is prevented and the birds develop a natural immunity as a result of being exposed to a mild infection.

Most poultry producers run this type of programme for about 14 weeks. Inherent in this system, despite its advantage, is the danger that low-level therapy will lead to the appearance of drug-resistant strains of coccidia.

(2) Some producers withhold treatment until signs of coccidiosis are recognized in the unit—this method depends on acute observation by the staff of the unit and failures can be expensive.

(3) A form of immunization is practised—three-day-old chicks are given measured quantities of the oocysts of up to seven different species of coccidia in the feed or drinking water. A mild infection is induced which allows the development of immunity. In addition, a low level of a coccidiostat may be used to prevent any accidental over-exposure to disease.

Plan 1 is obviously the simplest and safest.

With the range of coccidiostats which are now available it is possible, by switching treatments from time to time, to prevent the development of obvious drug resistance. The farmer needs, however, to be aware of the different modes of action of available coccidiostats so that any change of therapy offers a genuinely new form of preventive therapy.

Drug resistance

Reports of coccidia showing resistance to a coccidiostat invariably follow the introduction of a new drug. In some cases resistance has developed, but in others the incidence of disease has been found to be due to an intercurrent infection of coli septicaemia or fowl pest or the development to an infective level of a previously unrecognized species of coccidium. It is important, therefore, in the testing of a new drug to investigate the effect of artificially developed resistance to the drug and this is usually achieved by regularly passaging coccidia in birds in the presence of sub-optimal concentrations of the drug until resistance develops. It is important also to ensure that pure cultures of specific coccidia are maintained and that pathogen-free chicks are used so that it is possible to identify the cause of infection should it occur during the period of test.

Among the newer drugs it has not been found possible to demonstrate resistance to monensin or lasalocid even though over 20 passages have been carried out. In the case of monensin the failure to induce resistance may be due to the fact that monensin does not act directly on the parasite but may modify the host cell in a way that renders the environment unsuitable for the parasite to thrive. It is essential, however, if a new drug is to remain useful in the field that its use be monitored to ensure that false claims of resistance do not lead to the rejection of a valuable drug.

Major coccidiostats

The majority of effective coccidiostats show their greatest activity against the first or second asexual cycle and none has significant activity during the period of the sexual cycle. Little, however, is known about the chemical metabolic pathway by which a drug blocks the stage of development of the coccidia.

Table 8.1 gives an indication of the major coccidiostats used in poultry and their period of activity during an asexual cycle. In addition to the use of individual coccidiostats, a number of formulations include coccidiostat combinations, usually with a sulphonamide content (Table 8.2). Potentiated mixtures are rendered more effective than each individual drug alone by the fact that each drug in the combination acts on sequential steps in the enzymatic pathway by which micro-organisms synthesize tetrahydrofolate from precursor molecules.

Sulphonamides

The sulphonamides were the first drugs to have proven activity against coccidia and they were introduced for use in the period 1940–1948. They act

Table 8.1. Major anticoccidial drugs in order of their introduction for use.
Drugs are classified as coccidiocides (killing coccidia) or coccidiostats (inhibiting multiplication)
according to Cruthers and Szanto (1980).

Chemical activity	Generic name	Site and time of activity	Coccidiostat or coccidiocide
Sulphonamides	sulphanilamide		coccidiocide
	sulphaguanidine	Day 4, second	coccidiocide
	sulphamethazine	asexual cycle	coccidiocide
	sulphaquinoxaline		coccidiocide
	sulphanitron		coccidiocide
Nitrofurans	furazolidone		
	nitrofurazone		coccidiostat
Nitrophenide	nitrophenide	Day 4, second asexual cycle	coccidiostat
Carbanilides	nicarbazine	Day 4, second asexual cycle	both
Pyrimidine derivatives	amprolium ethopabate diaveridine pyrimethamine	Day 3, first asexual cycle	coccidiostat
Nitrobenzamide	zoalene (dinitolmide)	Day 3, second asexual cycle	both
4-Hydroxyquinolines	buquinolate decoquinate methylbenzoquate	Day 1, first asexual cycle	coccidiostat
Pyridinols	clopidol	Day 1, first asexual cycle	coccidiostat
Polyethers	monensin lasalocid	Day 2, first asexual cycle	both
Guanidines	robenidine	Day 2, first asexual cycle	both
Nucleoside	arprinocid	Asexual cycle	

Table 8.2. Coccidiostat combinations.

Trade name	Combinations	Anticoccidial use
Pancoxin	sulphaquinoxaline + amprolium + ethopabate	Prophylactic
Supracox	sulphaquinoxaline + amprolium + ethopabate + pyrimethamine	,,
Unistat	sulphanitran + nitromide + roxarsone	,,
Potentiated mixtures		
Whitsyns	sulphaquinoxaline + pyrimethamine	Prophylactic
Darvisul	sulphaquinoxaline + diaveridine	,,

as *p*-aminobenzoic acid antagonists, blocking the synthesis of the essential vitamin tetrahydrofolic acid. The earlier sulphonamides had limited value for the prevention of coccidiosis in poultry because when they had to be used for long periods, particularly at therapeutic levels, they caused severe haemorrhages in some of the treated chicks.

Sulphaquinoxaline proved to be the most active and is used on its own or, more frequently, in a number of combinations with amprolium, ethopabate or pyrimethamine.

Sulphaquinoxaline   Sulphamethazine

The sulphonamides are more effective against the intestinal coccidia rather than the important *E. tenella* which is found in the caeca. Their maximum effect is against the second-stage schizonts. The potentiated mixtures with ethopabate or pyrimethamine are uniquely effective in that they interfere with different phases of the *p*-aminobenzoic acid pathway.

Nitrofurans

The nitrofurans, such as furazolidone, were introduced as coccidiostats in 1948 and, although limited in action, had wide usage until superseded by nicarbazine and amprolium.

Furazolidone

Nitrophenide

This was one of the coccidiostats introduced in the early 1950s and it was active mainly against *E. tenella* which at the time was considered to be the main pathogen in chicken coccidiosis. It has now been replaced by more active chemicals.

Nicarbazin

Nicarbazin is an equimolecular complex of N,N'-di(*p*-nitrophenyl)urea (or dinitrocarbanilide—DNC) and 1-hydroxy-3,5-dimethylpyrimidine (HPD).

Nicarbazin was introduced in 1955 and was an advance in that it was active against *E. necatrix* and *E. acervulina* in addition to *E. tenella*. It had a

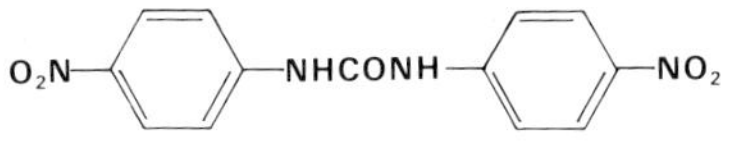

N,N'-di(*p*-nitrophenyl)urea 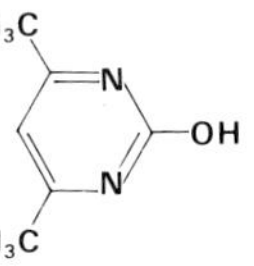   1-hydroxy-3,5-dimethylpyrimidine

toxic action in laying birds and can influence hatchability, so that its use latterly has been confined to broilers. Although still used for inclusion in broiler mashes, it has been largely superseded by the more effective modern coccidiostats.

Amprolium

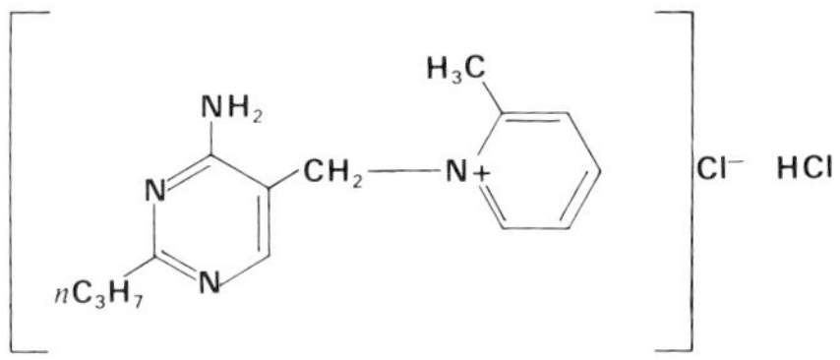

Amprolium was introduced in 1960 and is still in general use for the prevention of infection in replacement birds being kept for egg laying, and in layers. It is rarely used for broilers on its own because of its poor activity against *E. maxima* and *E. mivati*, and it is generally combined with ethopabate or other potentiators (see Table 8.1). It acts by mimicking thiamine in the metabolism of the parasite.

Ethopabate

Ethopabate is a substituted benzoic acid methyl ester.

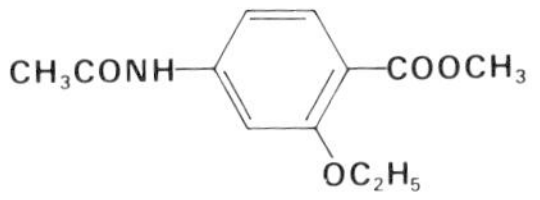

Ethopabate: methyl 2-ethoxy-4-acetamidobenzoate.

It is active against *E. maxima* and *E. brunetti* but has little activity against *E. tenella*, so it has found its main use in combination with amprolium and/or sulphaquinoxaline.

Zoalene

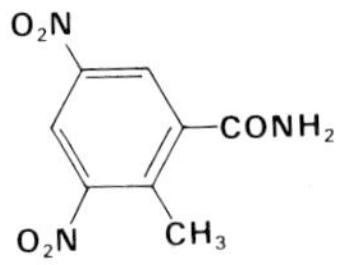

Zoalene: 2-methyl-3,5-dinitrobenzamide

Zoalene, as this chemical is generally known, is used largely as a preventive and its main action is against *E. tenella*, although as a preventive it also has some activity against *E. necatrix*, *E. acervulina* and *E. maxima*.

Quinolones

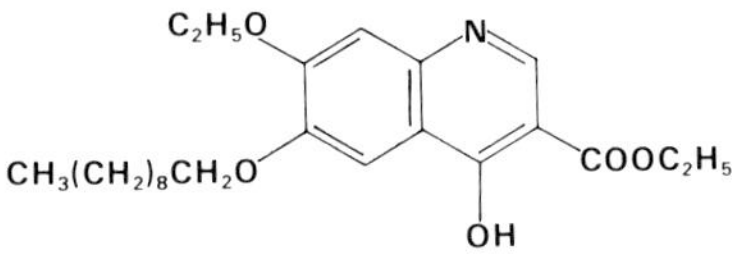

Decoquinate

The quinolones (buquinolate, decoquinate and methyl benzoquate), although highly active against coccidia and of low toxicity, had a relatively short life as major coccidiostats as they had a tendency to allow drug-resistant strains to develop. They are still occasionally used when rapid withdrawal of a feed is necessary and resistance would not be of significance.

Clopidol

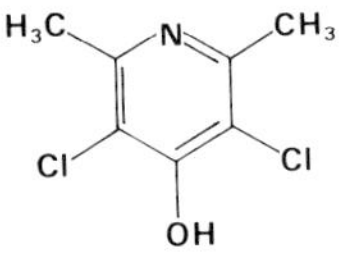

Clopidol is active at the earliest stage of development of a coccidium (the sporozoite), so that it can be used only as a preventive. Because of this early effect, little immunity to coccidia is developed within the treated chicks, so that clopidol is mainly of value for broilers where it can be given throughout the life of the chick to slaughter.

Monensin

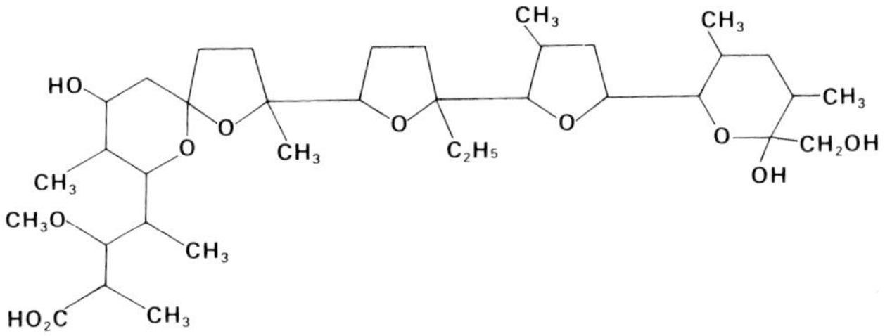

Monensin, unlike its predecessors, is a natural product produced by fermentation and is recovered from *Streptomyces cinnamonensis*. Its anticoccidial action occurs during the first two days of the life cycle, against the schizont stage of the parasite. It forms complexes (ionophores) in the host and in the parasite. This affects the sodium and potassium ions, leading to an interference in the development of the parasite. The fact that the chemical produces ionophore complexes in the host as well as the parasite means that overdosage has to be avoided.

Monensin has proved to be a very effective coccidiostat against all the major strains and it is difficult to initiate resistance under experimental conditions.

Lasalocid

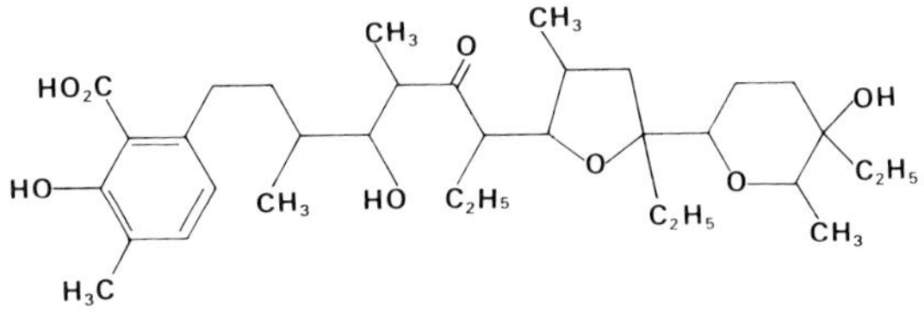

Lasalocid is produced from the fermentation of *Streptomyces lasaliensis* and has a similar range of anticoccidial activity to monensin. It produces complexes (ionophores) but they are different from those formed by monensin, and it can combine with both monovalent and divalent cations. It is used mainly for the control of coccidiosis in broilers.

Robenidine

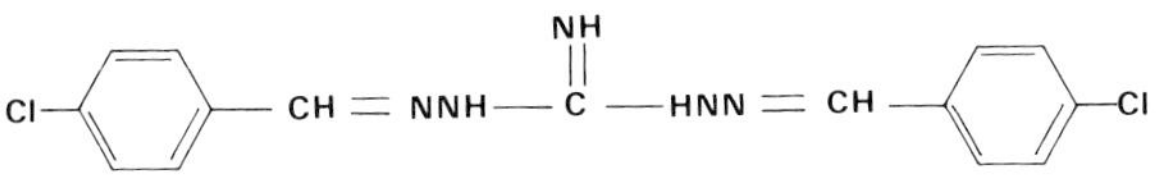

In laboratory experiments robenidine is very effective against the major coccidia and proved to be a very effective coccidiostat when first introduced. Drug resistance, however, occurred at a relatively early stage, so that the drug is not now widely used. In addition, it gave an unpleasant taste to parts of the flesh of broilers.

It acts by preventing the differentiation of merozoites to form mature schizonts.

Arprinocid

This is a broad-spectrum coccidiostat and is an analogue of a nucleoside. It acts at the asexual stage of the life cycle and, in addition, interferes with the sporulation of the oocyst. Within the parasite it acts on purine metabolism and the parent drug is converted to an active form *in vivo*.

Coccidial infections in animals other than poultry

Coccidiosis also occurs in turkeys and game birds and the infections respond to many of the chemicals which have been introduced for the prevention of infection in poultry. Because turkeys are not kept as intensively as poultry and the infection may not be as severe, many of the coccidiostats can be used therapeutically in turkey houses. At the present time sulphaquinoxaline, furazolidone, amprolium and zoalene are all used for coccidiosis control in turkeys.

Cattle and sheep can also carry a wide range of coccidia—up to 12 different species have been recorded throughout the world. However, control and treatment are applied only sporadically, as the condition is seldom recognized as a single problem and any infection is often associated with other causal agents such as *Salmonella* and frequently *E. coli*. Ideally, where coccidiosis is recognized in cattle and sheep it should be treated preventively, as therapy of established infections is not very effective. If coccidia are considered to be the major causal organism of disease, preventive therapy should be instituted on a regular basis until the infection is eliminated. Sulphamethazine, amprolium and monensin are used in these animals.

Table 8.3. Protozoa and bacteria spread by ticks and causing disease in cattle.

Disease	Causal organism	Transmitting ticks	World distribution
Anaplasmosis (gall sickness)	*Anaplasma marginale*	*Boophilus* spp. *Dermacentor* spp. *Rhipicephalus* spp.	Asia, Australia, Africa, North, Central and South America, Mediterranean countries
Piroplasmosis (tick fever)	*Babesia bigemina* *B. argentina* *B. bovis*	*Boophilus* spp. *Rhipicephalus* spp. *Ixodes ricinus*	Asia, Australia, Africa, North, Central and South America, West Indies, Europe
Heartwater	Rickettsiae (minute rod-shaped bacteria)	*Amblyomma* spp.	East, Central and South Africa
Theileriosis (East Coast fever)	*Theileria* spp.	*Rhipicephalus* spp.	East Africa – Kenya, Uganda, Tanzania
(a) Tropical disease	*Theileria annulata*	*Hyalomma* spp.	Southern Asia, North Africa, Southern Europe
(b) Australian theileriosis	*Theileria mutans*	*Haemophalis longicornis*	Australia

Table 8.4. Protozoa spread by tsetse fly and tabanids (blood-sucking flies).

Disease	Causal organism	Transmitting fly	World distribution
Trypanosomiasis	*T. brucei* *T. vivax* *T. congolense*	Tsetse fly Tabanids	East and West Africa (cattle)
Trypanosomiasis	*T. evansi*	Tabanids	Sudan (camels)
Trypanosomiasis	*T. equiperdum* *T. equinum*	Tabanids	South America (horses)

Other protozoal diseases

Protozoa other than coccidia can cause a wide range of diseases in animals and the majority of the diseases are spread by either ticks or blood-sucking insects (Tables 8.3 and 8.4).

A number of chemicals have been developed over the last fifty years to deal specifically with babesia, anaplasma and trypanosome infections. However, unless technical support from FAO or WHO and financial support from the World Bank become available, it is unlikely that the major research projects necessary to discover and test new chemicals will be initiated by the

Table 8.5.   Chemicals used in the therapy of tropical protozoal and bacterial diseases.

Infecting organisms	Disease	Chemical
Anaplasma	Anaplasmosis	Imidocarb, tetracyclines
Babesia bigemina	Texas fever	Amicarbalide, imidocarb
B. bovis	Red water fever	Diminazene, imidocarb
B. argentina	Red water fever	Phenamidine, imidocarb Quinuronium
Rickettsiae	Heartwater	Tetracyclines
Theileria spp.	Theileriosis (East coast fever)	
Trypanosoma brucei	Trypanosomiasis	Homidium, quinapyramine
T. vivax	Trypanosomiasis	Diminazene
T. congolense	Nagana	Diminazene, homidium
T. evansi	Surra	Suramin, quinapyramine
T. equiperdum	Dourine	Suramin
T. equinum	Mal de caderas	Suramin

pharmaceutical companies, as the return on the investment could not be guaranteed. A description is given now of the major chemical groups used in this field.

Antipiroplasma compounds

Because of the wide range of the babesia species which can infect cattle, horses and dogs, it is essential that the full range of drugs described should be available for use. The aim in therapy is to reduce the number of parasites present in the blood so that an immunity to the infection is developed. Where prophylaxis is practised it is often used in association with an immunization programme. Imidocarb in particular is given before inoculation of small doses of blood from carrier animals.

All the antipiroplasma drugs can produce toxic reactions and this is associated particularly with repeat therapeutic treatment. This effect is not surprising in view of the known binding of the drugs to plasma and the liver and kidneys.

Resistance can occur to all the existing drugs but the extent of resistance is unknown.

Diminazene

Mode of action

The drug has an effect on glycolysis and this leads to hypoglycaemia in the treated animal. There is also a selective blocking of kinetoplast DNA replication (Newton 1970). The drug is irreversibly bound by the DNA of a trypanosome although this has not been demonstrated conclusively in babesia.

Pharmacokinetics

The action of diminazene on protozoa appears to be due to its persistence in the body, as following injection only transient levels of drug are found in the plasma. The chemical, however, accumulates in the liver and kidneys and remains there for several months. In this way a therapeutic and prophylactic effect against infection can occur.

Usage

Because of the binding of diminazene to the liver and kidney tissues, the drug should, where possible, be given to the animal prior to infection. This prophylactic use is of value when a tick-free animal is being moved through a tick-infested area.

Phenamidine isethionate

Phenamidine isethionate is 4,4'-diamidinodiphenyl ether di-(β-hydroxyethane sulphonate).

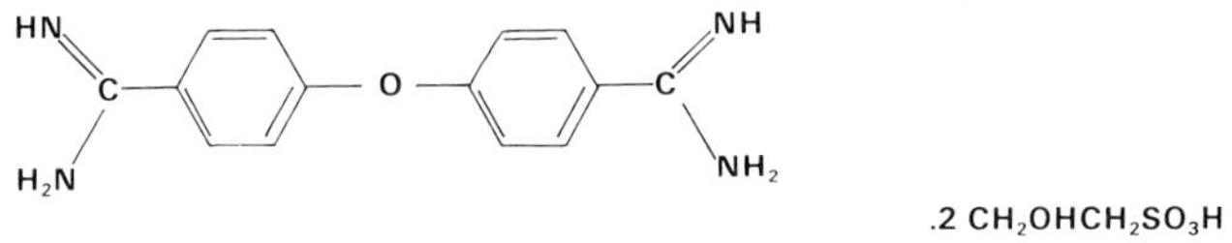

.2 CH$_2$OHCH$_2$SO$_3$H

The mode of action of phenamidine is similar to that of diminazene and is related to persistence in the body and the action on the DNA of the parasite.

Amicarbalide isethionate

Amicarbalide isethionate is 3,3'-diamidinocarbanilide di-isethionate.

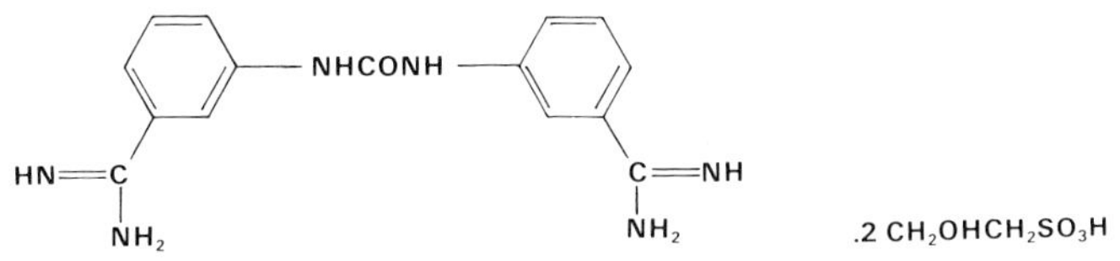

.2 CH$_2$OHCH$_2$SO$_3$H

Amicarbalide has a similar pharmacology and mode of action to the two preceding chemicals.

Imidocarb dipropionate

Imidocarb dipropionate is 3,3-bis-(2-imidazolin-2-yl)carbanilide dipropionate.

2 CH₃CH₂COOH

Originally imidocarb proved toxic in use but work by Aliu *et al.* (1977) reported that 2 mg/kg bodyweight imidocarb given intravenously to a sheep produced a peak level of 10·8 mg/ml which dropped rapidly to 1·9 mg/ml within an hour. The drug was found to be bound to plasma and other tissues for over four weeks when given intramuscularly, and did not produce any toxic reaction. The mode of action is similar to that of the previously mentioned drugs.

Anaplasmosis

Because of the importance of this disease in tropical countries, treatment has to be carried out to prevent the development of large numbers of carrier animals. Both the antibiotic oxytetracycline and amidocarb are used for treatment. Oxytetracycline as a long-acting injection is used in cattle at a dose of 20 mg/kg at intervals of a week (Roby *et al.* 1978). Imidocarb is recommended at a dose of 3 mg/kg.

Trypanosomiasis

Trypanosome infections spread by tsetse flies are confined to certain areas of East and West Africa where the environment favours the survival of the tsetse fly. Because the attack of a tsetse fly cannot be predicted, the aim with anti-trypanosome treatment is to achieve a prophylactic effect so that the drug will be present in the body when the trypanosome first enters the blood.

A number of chemicals have been introduced for use since the early 1950s and all have had failures when resistant trypanosome strains have been found in the blood. Four groups of drugs are still in use in Africa: (1) phenanthridines (homidium, pyrithidium, isometamidium), (2) suramin, (3) quinapyramine (Antrycide), (4) diminazene (Berenil).

Homidium bromide (Novidium)

Homidium bromide is 2,7-diamino-9-phenyl-10-ethylphenanthridinium and belongs to the group of drugs described as phenanthridines.

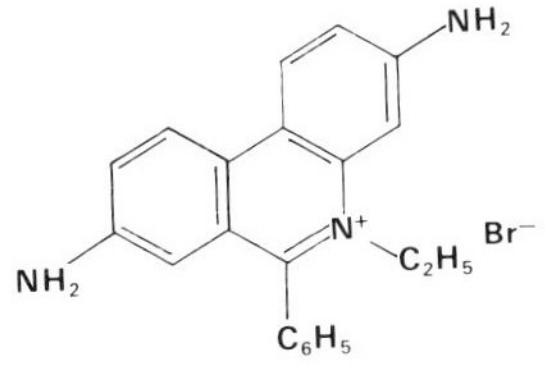

Mode of action

Its action is dependent on its ability to bind strongly to nucleic acids, especially the DNA of the parasite. Details of this action are discussed by Klein (1980), both as it relates to a number of the drugs used for prophylaxis and treatment of such protozoa as babesia and trypanosomes.

Usage

It is used at a dose of 1 mg/kg bodyweight and is given intramuscularly; a single treatment has both a curative and prophylactic effect. Like other effective antiprotozoal drugs, homidium persists in the body but it is now considered that the main use should be as a curative drug, as the prophylactic effect is of value only where there is a low risk of tsetse attack.

Toxicology

Local reactions which sometimes follow subcutaneous injection can be reduced by deep intramuscular injection.

Pyrithidium (Prothidium) and isometamidium (Samorin)

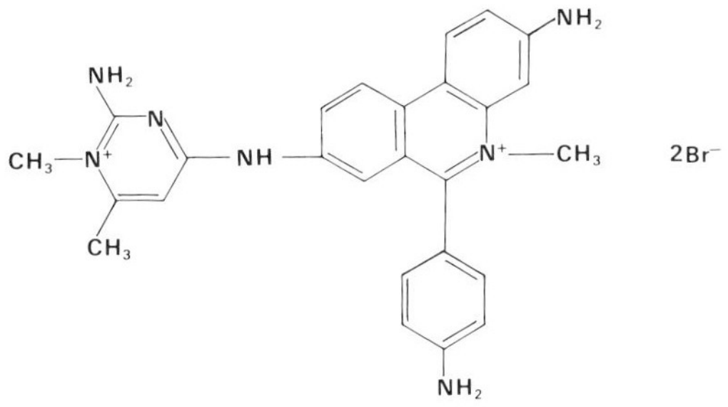

Pyrithidium

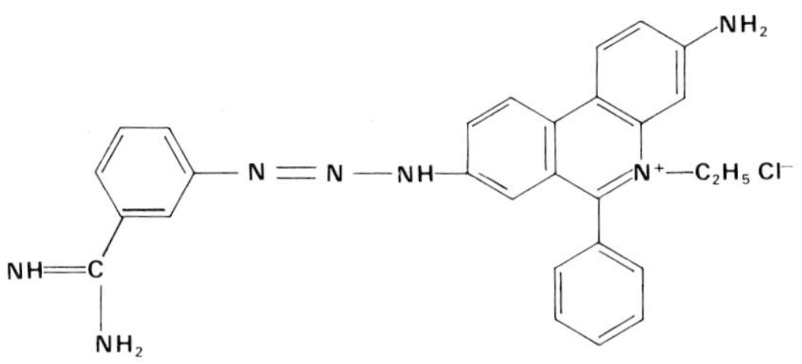

Isometamidium

Both these drugs have very similar actions to homidium and both bind to the nucleic acids of the parasites. They are used for curative and prophylactic effects.

Suramin

Suramin is the symmetrical 3″-urea of the sodium salt of 8-(3-benzamido-4-methylbenzamido)naphthalene-1,3,5-tri-sulphonic acid. It is known to inhibit a number of enzyme systems within the parasite, including ATPases and glycerophosphate oxidase, but its exact mode of action has not been established. It is now mainly used in animals for the cure of *T. evansi* infections. It can also be used for *T. equinum* (mal de caderas) and *T. equiperdum* (dourine) in horses.

Suramin has a low safety margin in horses, so has to be given with care.

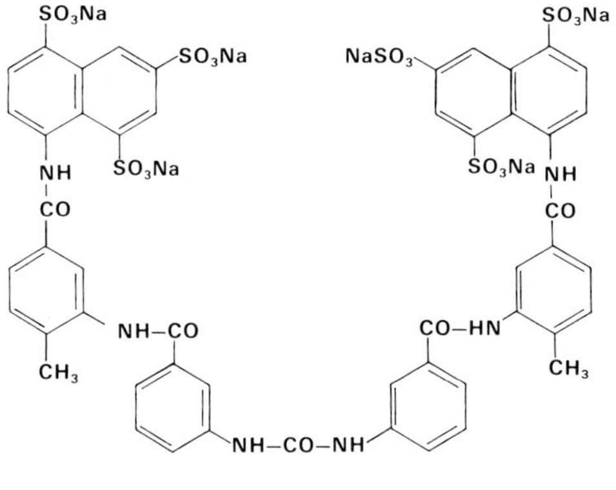

Suramin

Quinapyramines

Two salts of quinapyramine, chloride and sulphate, are used for the control of trypanosomiasis. The chloride is slowly absorbed and acts prophylactically, whereas the sulphate is absorbed rapidly and has a curative action.

Quinapyramine chloride

Quinapyramine chloride is 4-amino-6-(2-amino-6-methylpyrimid-4-yl-amino)-2-methylquinoline 1,1'-dimethochloride dihydrate, while the sulphate is the corresponding 1,1'-dimetho(methyl sulphate).

Mode of action

Quinpyramine binds to DNA and interferes with the incorporation of purines into nucleic acid, thus hindering the growth of the trypanosome. This effect can be demonstrated experimentally but the exact range of action in the living animal is not known.

Pharmacokinetics

The two chemicals have different actions because the sulphate salt is water-soluble and is readily absorbed, so has a rapid action in the body. The chloride salt is practically insoluble in water (up to 2%), so it is absorbed slowly when given by injection and acts as a depot drug, releasing the active principle over a relatively long period. Decisions on the use of the salts are based on local knowledge of tsetse fly activity and the incidence of acute infections.

Toxicology

Reactions can occur in individual animals following dosage, but they are usually of a transient nature.

9. Growth promoters

Introduction

Growth promoters are substances which are not nutrients in their own right but, when given in small quantities regularly in the feed or by implant, have an effect which leads to an increase in growth rate and/or feed conversion efficiency in animals fed a diet which is nutritionally adequate. The major growth promoters used in animal production are antibiotics or antibacterials, hormone implants which are usually mixtures of natural or synthetically produced hormone preparations, and a third category of growth promoter which acts specifically in the rumen of cattle and sheep by improving rumen activity and the availability of propionic acid.

Antibacterials

The oral antibacterial growth promoters are most widely used as additions to the feed of poultry and pigs, and the majority of those used have large molecules; their action takes place in the lumen of the gut, as the larger molecules are unlikely to have been absorbed intact. Although still debated, it is generally considered that the growth effect is achieved by the action of the antibacterials on the microflora (or their products) present in the gastro-intestinal lumen, so that the efficiency of carbohydrate and nitrogen digestion is enhanced. The average gain from antibacterial growth promoters has remained relatively constant over the last 25 years, so that it appears that the effect on gut bacteria is unrelated to antibiotic resistance or transfer of resistance from organism to organism.

In the early 1950s (Coates *et al.* 1955) it was shown that very small quantities of penicillin (10 g to 1 ton of feed) led to a marked increase in the growth of chicks and it was subsequently demonstrated that the increased growth achieved was similar to that shown when chicks were kept in a germ-free environment. Since that time most new antibiotics have been examined for their value in stimulating increased growth in poultry and pigs kept on a standard diet. The response is normally greatest in simple-stomached animals such as poultry and pigs. By the early 1960s penicillin, tetracyclines, chloramphenicol and neomycin were all used as growth promoters, in some cases in increasing doses.

During this period also, the medical and veterinary profession became aware that the increase in resistant bacterial strains, found both during human and animal treatment, was becoming a major problem in the control of some infections. In the UK, a committee of investigation, the Swann Committee, was appointed to advise on the use of antibiotics and antibacterials for the treatment and prevention of disease in animals. The committee was able to recommend that, although there was a possible link between the human and animal therapy of bacterial diseases, it was not proven that the treatment of clinical diseases in animals with antibiotics would reduce the value of these drugs for human use. It was agreed, however, that only certain antibiotics and antibacterials which were little used for human therapy should be defined as growth promoters. These growth promoters could be included in the feed of poultry and pigs at certain clearly defined levels.

There are now about 20 antibacterial agents which can promote growth in one or more species. Further information on this subject can be found in Visek (1978).

Control of growth promoter use

The EEC controls the use of growth promoters and has issued a directive which lists antibacterials which may be used for growth promotion. In EEC countries, if a medicinal product such as an antibiotic is included in a feed at a growth promotion level, it is described as an *additive*, whereas the term *medicated feed* is used to describe any mixture of one or more veterinary medicinal products and one or more feeding stuffs which is prepared prior to sale for use as a prophylactic or therapeutic feed stuff.

A simple method of considering the use of antibacterials in the feed is as follows.

Low level addition 5–15 parts/10^6	— to improve growth rate in apparently healthy animals.
Medium level addition 50–150 parts/10^6	— to prevent infectious disease in animals under stress.
High level addition 350–1000 parts/10^6	— to treat *diseased* animals.

In the USA, comprehensive feed compendia are published each year which describe the drugs which may legally be added to the feed of cattle, pigs and poultry. These compendia are very detailed and cover both additives and medicated feeds and in addition to describing the specific feed additive, for example Bacitracin, indicate the species of animal which may be treated,

Table 9.1. Major growth promoters which are not absorbed.

Compound	Class	Source	Spectrum of activity	Class of animal treated
Avoparcin	antibiotic	*Streptomyces candidus*	Gram-positive	poultry
Flavomycin	antibiotic	*Streptomyces bambergiensis*	Gram-positive	poultry
Halquinol	chlorinated quinolinol	Synthetic	Broad spectrum	pigs
Nitrovin	nitrofuran	Synthetic	Gram-positive	poultry
Thiopeptin	antibiotic	*Streptomyces lateyamensis*	Gram-positive	pigs
Virginiamycin	antibiotic	*Streptomyces virginiae*	Gram-positive	poultry
Zinc bacitracin	antibiotic	*B licheniformis*	Gram-positive	poultry

Table 9.2. Major growth promoters which are absorbed.

Compound	Class	Source	Spectrum of activity	Class of animal treated
Arsanilic acid	arsenical	Synthetic	Non-specific	pigs
Carbadox	quinoxaline NN-dioxide derivative	Synthetic	Broad-spectrum	pigs
Tylosin	antibiotic	*Streptomyces fradiae*	Gram-positive, *Mycoplasma* and *Treponema*	pigs
Tiamulin	antibiotic	*Pleurotus mutilis*	Gram-positive, *Mycoplasma* and *Treponema*	pigs
Mupirocin	antibiotic	*Pseudomonas fluorescens*	Gram-positive, some Gram-negative, and *Treponema*	pigs

the approved dose level, and the claims that may be made for the effects of therapy. New tables are published each year to allow for additions or removals when new information becomes available.

Tables 9.1 and 9.2 give lists of antibiotics and antibacterials which are commonly used as growth promoters. It will be noted that the majority are not absorbed from the gut.

Certain other chemicals such as copper and cobalt salts are used as growth promoters. Copper is added to the feed of young pigs to counter the enteritis which frequently occurs, and it has been demonstrated also to have a growth promotion effect of its own. In addition, copper and cobalt are added to the feed or given orally or parenterally to counter recognized mineral deficiencies which can affect the growth of sheep and cattle.

Anabolic agents

It has been common practice throughout the world to castrate male cattle which are to be kept for fattening. It was found that the animals became more docile and management of the cattle in groups was greatly simplified.

The removal of the testes however, led to the loss of the secretion of the androgen steroids, in particular, testosterone. The lack of the hormones tended to slow down growth, reduced feed conversion efficiency and also led to a fatter carcase. To counter this effect, and still have the beneficial effect of ease of handling, hormones or anabolic agents were designed for implantation in castrated animals and their presence in the body countered the adverse effect of castration.

It was also found that anabolic agents could be used to good effect in increasing growth rate in heifers, cows and bulls. Anabolic agents can increase feed conversion efficiency, the lean content of the tissues, and growth rate in animals because of their ability to increase nitrogen retention and protein deposition.

In 1981, because of the recognized adverse effects of certain synthetic oestrogens such as stilboestrol and hexoestrol which were generally used as implants, the anabolic agents which were in use as growth promoters were reviewed and only the natural hormones oestradiol, progesterone and testosterone were approved for use in the EEC. They were considered safe because they are normally present in the body. Two other substances—a synthetic steroid, trenbolone, and a synthetic oestrogen, zeranol—were also approved because of their demonstrated safety.

Oestrogens

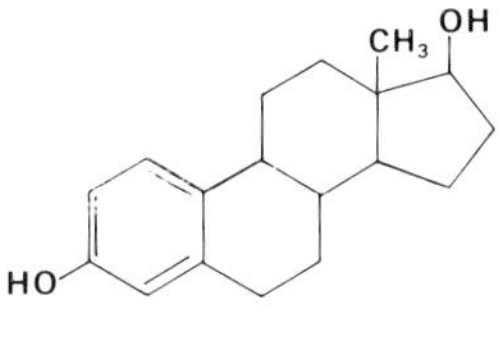

Oestradiol

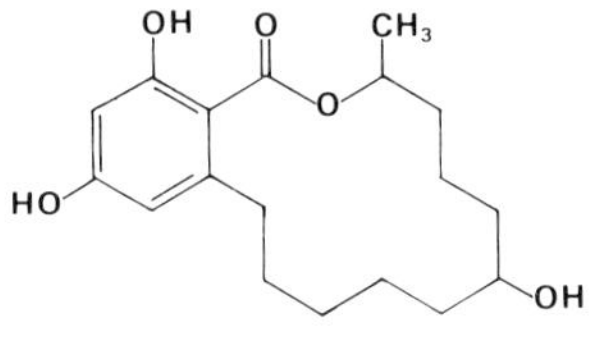

Zeranol

Androgen

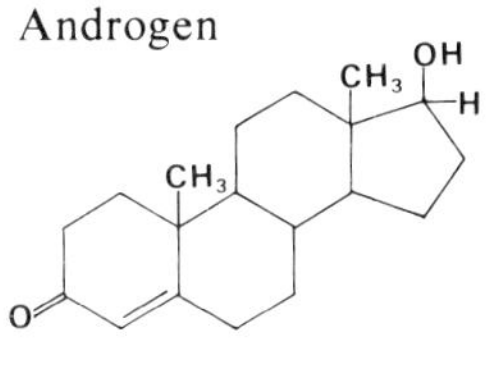

Testosterone

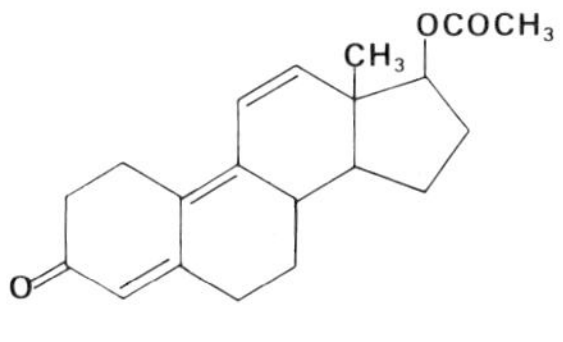

Trenbolone acetate

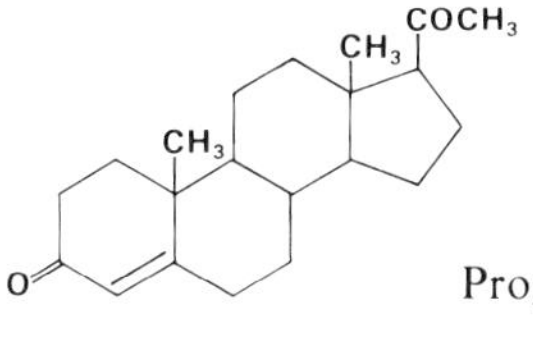

Progesterone

Table 9.3. Anabolic growth promoters—dosage level and withdrawal period.

Anabolic agent	Animal to be treated	Dosage	Withdrawal period
Trenbolone acetate	Heifers, calves and cull cows	300 mg	60 days
Zeranol	Steers, calves and wether lambs	36 mg	70 days
Oestradiol + progesterone	Steers	O: 20 mg P: 200 mg	0 days
Testosterone + oestradiol	Heifers and cull cows	T: 200 mg O: 20 mg	0 days
Oestradiol + progesterone	Male veal calves	O: 20 mg P: 200 mg	90 days
Testosterone + oestradiol	Female veal calves	T: 200 mg O: 20 mg	90 days

The anabolic agents are formulated as pellets for subcutaneous implant at the back of the ear. The agents are slowly released and have the effect of supplementing the sex steroids already present in the body.

Table 9.3 indicates the dosage rates recommended for anabolic growth promoters and the recommended withdrawal periods.

The maximum growth stimulation is achieved when both androgen and oestrogen are circulating in the blood at levels normally found in uncastrated bulls or cows.

Mode of action

Plasma concentrations of growth hormone from the anterior pituitary gland and insulin are increased when oestrogens are used—this stimulates amino-acid uptake into muscles. The androgens, such as testosterone, appear to reduce the breakdown of proteins.

Both androgens and oestrogens are necessary to achieve maximum growth rates in ruminants. Because of this, the exogenous hormone provided by an implant supplements the hormone already existing in the body. The most successful responses are obtained in heifers and cows treated with androgens, and steers and veal calves receiving combined preparations of androgen and oestrogen.

Growth responses of up to 40% gain have been reported from the use of these growth promoters, so they are used by most farmers who fatten cattle.

Residues

Residues of anabolic agents in treated animals are detected by radiometric techniques, and at the slaughterhouse the lowest levels can be detected by the use of radio-immuno-assays. It has also been found that approximately 10–20% of the original dose implanted in the ears is there at slaughter, so removal of the ear is absolutely vital. When used under recommended conditions, the residues in meat are 1–2 orders of magnitude lower than those which occur naturally in bulls and pregnant cows.

Human safety

The three natural steroids, oestradiol, testosterone and progesterone are naturally present in humans and animals in concentrations which are higher than any likely level which would follow from eating meat of implanted animals.

Improvement in ruminal efficiency

The third area of growth promotion is that of improving the ruminal digestive action in ruminants. The ability of cattle, sheep and goats to digest relatively coarse fibres such as straw, hay or grass by means of fermentation in the rumen (one of the four stomachs) has always made these species valuable. But grass on its own has never been sufficient to sustain the modern cow, which is expected to carry a calf annually and to produce ever-increasing amounts of milk, or as a steer to produce a finished carcase in a year. The discovery that monensin, a polyether antibiotic originally used only as a coccidiostat (see page 125), was able to shift the balance of volatile fatty acids in the rumen towards increased propionic acid production was a considerable advance. Propionic acid enhances an animal's ability to use carbohydrate so that the use of monensin in the feed when the animal's diet was largely either grass-based or grain led to an improvement in growth performance.

When animals are housed, 20–40 p.p.m. (=20–40 g/ton) monensin is included in the feed, whereas animals at pasture receive 200 mg monensin per head.

Since the original work on monensin was published, several new chemicals have been added to the list of growth promoters which have a beneficial effect on rumen fermentation. These are:

  lasalocid—an ionophore like monensin;
  virginiamycin—an antibiotic used for growth promotion in poultry;
  avoparcin—an antibiotic used for growth promotion in poultry;
  nararsin and salinomycin.

Conclusion

The range of growth promoters which are available for all aspects of animal production perform a vital function in animal rearing by increasing food conversion efficiency and reducing the time taken for animals to reach the market. This has a marked effect on the amount of cereal used worldwide for animal production.

10. Hormones

Introduction

Hormones are messenger substances which stimulate activity in various organs of the body. The word is derived from the Greek and means 'to stimulate or urge on'. Hormones are secreted in small quantities and yet exert profound effects. They act quickly, although not as quickly as a nerve impulse.

Hormones are secreted by a number of glands which form the endocrine system, one of the two control systems of the body (pituitary, ovary, testes, adrenal glands, pancreas, thyroid, kidney and uterus). The endocrine glands differ from other glands (such as salivary glands) because they secrete their active principle directly into the bloodstream. Hormones can have a very specific activity (for example, insulin in carbohydrate metabolism) or may have a generalized action (for example, adrenalin in the fight/flight reflex).

Hormones belong to three classes of chemical compounds.

(1) *Amines, peptides and proteins*. Hormones of this type originate in the brain (e.g. in the pituitary gland), the thyroid and parathyroid glands, the adrenal glands and the kidney.

(2) *Steroids*. Hormones of this type are formed primarily in adrenals, ovaries and testes.

(3) *Fatty acids*. Hormones of this type include the prostaglandins which are found in many tissues but those of particular relevance to animal treatment are secreted by the uterus.

Hormone therapy is a complex subject and forms a very important aspect of veterinary medicine. The profitability of breeding herds and flocks relies on efficient reproduction. Frequently individual animals require hormonal therapy to improve their fertility. Group treatment is now also very important for synchronizing oestrus in sheep and cattle to facilitate artificial insemination, using progestins and prostaglandins, and for the induction of parturition using corticosteroids and prostaglandins. For dogs and cats, sex hormone therapy provides an alternative to surgery for controlling the nuisance of regular oestrus in bitches and cats, and for correcting aberrant sexual behaviour in dogs (progestins).

Table 10.1.   Chemical structures of hormones.

Amines, peptides and proteins
Example: Thyroxin—the active secretion of the thyroid gland.

Steroids
Example: Progesterone—secreted by the ovary.

Fatty acids—Prostaglandins
Example: prostanoic acid—parent compound of prostaglandins.

The protein/peptide hormones

The hormones of this type are produced by the anterior pituitary gland which is situated below the brain, and also by the human and equine placenta. These hormones are called gonadotrophins because they have a direct stimulating effect on the sex organs in males and females. The gonadotrophins are the same in the male and female—Follicle Stimulating Hormone (FSH) and Luteinizing Hormone (LH). In the male they stimulate the production of the male sex hormone (testosterone) and control the development and production of sperm. In the female, FSH and LH stimulate the production of oestrogen by the developing ovarian follicle, and of progesterone by the corpus luteum (a mass of endocrine cells present in the ruptured Graafian follicle of the ovary, which is formed after the release of the ovum). The gonadotrophins are essential for controlling the changes which take place during the reproductive cycle.

The gonadotrophins are proteins and are too complex to synthesize economically, and for the same reason they are not extracted from brain tissue. Fortunately there are naturally occurring alternatives:

Human chorionic gonadotrophin (HCG). This is prepared from the urine of pregnant women. It has FSH and LH activity. It is used as a luteinizing agent to induce ovulation at breeding time, particularly in mares and cows. It is also used to induce ovulation and luteinization in cattle with cystic ovaries. It may also be used in repeated small doses to stimulate ovarian activity in all species.

Human menopausal gonadotrophin (HMG). This is prepared from the urine of post-menopausal women and has essentially follicle stimulating activity.

Pregnant mare serum gonadotrophin (PMSG). In veterinary medicine PMSG is preferred to HMG. PMSG is produced by the equine placenta between the 50th and 80th days of pregnancy. The extract is prepared from the mares' serum. It has both FSH and LH properties. PMSG is used to stimulate follicle growth in acyclical animals, but its most important use is to super-ovulate sheep and cattle to increase the numbers of twins born. As in women, the results are variable and unpredictable. Frequently triplets, quadruplets and quintuplets are born rather than twins. PMSG is now widely used for super-ovulating donor cattle and sheep before embryo transfer.

An alternative to this approach is the use of gonadotrophin-releasing hormones. These are small peptides which can be economically synthesized. They have the advantage of ensuring that the release of FSH and LH from the treated animal is in physiological quantities and proportions.

The steroid hormones

These are often called the sex hormones because they are produced by the ovary in females (oestrogen and progesterone) and by the testes in males (testosterone). The role of the sex hormones is shown in Table 10.2. Steroid hormones seldom circulate in the bloodstream in a pure chemical form. They are usually bound to specific carrier proteins (sex hormone binding globulins). Binding helps to prolong their action; even so the half-life of these hormones is short.

The naturally occurring sex hormones are comparatively simple to synthesize. However, they are not active when given by mouth. Striking advances have been made in the biological activity and oral absorption of synthetic derivatives, particularly those related to progesterone (progestins). Progesterone itself is used in implants to maintain pregnancy in animals prone to habitual abortion. Progestins are also used by implant or by intravaginal pessary to control the breeding cycle or synchronize oestrus to facilitate artificial insemination. Using progesterone and/or progestin treatment, sheep can

Table 10.2. Sex hormone produced specifically by the functional parts of the reproductive system.

Gland	Hormone	Functions and effects in the animal
Ovary	Oestroegens	(a) Development and maintenance of the cyclic changes which occur in the genital tract (b) Development of secondary sexual characteristics, and accessory sex organs (c) Development of duct system of the mammary gland and uterus
	Progesterone	(a) Assists in the development of the uterus in preparation for implantation of the ovum and in the maintenance of pregnancy (b) Stimulates mammary development
Testes	Testosterone	(a) Development of accessory sex organs and secondary sex characteristics; spermatogenesis

be induced to breed earlier in the summer so that more lambs can be sold for the Easter lamb market in Europe. In pet dogs, oestrogen is given by injection to prevent unwanted pregnancy in bitches. The treatment is very effective provided that the bitch is treated as soon as possible after mating. An oral progestin treatment—medroxy progesterone acetate—is available and is widely used in dogs and cats for completely suppressing oestrus or postponing it to a more convenient time.

Fatty acid hormones

The naturally occurring prostaglandin $F_{2\alpha}$ and the potent synthetic analogues, cloprostenol and fluprostenol, have been recent successful additions to veterinary therapy. They are luteolytic substances capable of causing premature regression of the corpus luteum in pregnant and non-pregnant animals.

Fluprostenol sodium

Prostaglandin is effective in mares and is used to induce ovarian activity caused by retention of the corpus luteum. It is also used as an aid to stud management to ensure that mares are in oestrus when presented to the stallion. In cattle, prostaglandins are used to synchronize oestrus and so facilitate artificial insemination; to induce abortion in the case of unwanted pregnancies and to treat cases of pyometra, mummified foetus and luteal ovarian cysts. Prostaglandin can also be used in cattle and pigs to induce calving and farrowing.

It is usual now to use HCG and PMS where a specific stimulation of ovulation is considered necessary, and the activity of the prostaglandin cloprostenol sodium as a luteolytic agent has provided a practical method of ensuring that the cows in a dairy herd come into oestrus approximately 50–60 days after calving. Trials over the last four years in dairy herds have demonstrated that by the use of cloprostenol (Estrumate) it is possible to maintain an efficient breeding programme in the majority of cows.

The first step towards the control of reproduction in both dairy and beef cattle was the development of artificial insemination. It made possible the selection of suitable males—the semen of one bull can now sire over 100 000 offspring in a year as compared with fifty by natural mating. If the benefits of artificial insemination are to be applied to the dairy herd as a whole, it is essential that the reproduction cycle of a cow is maintained in a way that ensures that insemination is followed by successful conception and the maintenance of pregnancy.

Cloprostenol—its use in dairy herds

Cloprostenol is structurally related to prostaglandin $F_{2\alpha}$ and is prepared in the form of an aqueous solution, each millilitre of which contains 236 μg of cloprostenol sodium which is given by intramuscular injection.

Mode of action

Cloprostenol acts as a luteolytic agent—it causes functional and morphological regression of the corpus luteum. The endocrine cells of the corpus luteum secrete the hormone progesterone which is responsible for the maintenance of pregnancy. Until the corpus luteum is luteolysed it is not possible to restart the process of oestrus which then leads to ovulation.

Use

Cloprostenol is used in dairy herds (*a*) to synchronize oestrus in a group of cows or (*b*) to control oestrus in an individual cow or (*c*) to facilitate the use of artificial insemination in a group of heifers. ICI has developed a series of programmes for the use of cloprostenol in dairy herds which ensure that artificial insemination is used effectively and that the calving index of the herd is maintained at an economic level. (The calving index refers to the period of gestation (280 days) plus the days to the next conception. Ideally the latter should be about 85 days, so the index is 365 days. This allows for a period of recovery from the pregnancy and also ensures that milk production will be maintained.)

The economic significance of maintaining a good calving index is demonstrated by the fact that peak milk yield occurs when the interval from calving to first service is between 41 and 48 days. If the interval is less than 35 days or more than 76 days, the milk yield will drop. Time of first service can be controlled by the use of cloprostenol.

Cloprostenol is also used for the control of a number of reproductive problems:

(1) treatment of cows, particularly heavy-yielding cows, which do not show obvious signs of oestrus;

(2) removal of unwanted pregnancies;

(3) removal of mummified foetuses;

(4) induction of parturition—within approximately 10 days or less of the predicted parturition date.

Conclusions

Veterinary endocrinology, particularly in the use of the sex hormones for the control of reproduction, has progressed very rapidly in recent years. Hormone therapy has an important part to play in maintaining the health and productivity of farm animals and in controlling the sexual cycle of pet animals. Hormones are potent substances which should only be used under the supervision of a veterinary surgeon if animals are to be protected from misuse and the public are to be protected from hormonal residues in meat and milk.

11. Legal control and testing for safety

UK legislation

The effective control of drugs for veterinary use in the UK followed the passing of the Medicines Act (1968) which established the standard of controls on the safety, quality, efficacy and supply of both medical and veterinary drugs. Before the introduction of this Act, voluntary controls had been applied to safety, quality and clinical testing and in some cases the route of sale, and these had proved to be very effective. However, as legislation became stricter in the USA, it was appreciated that standard practices for drug control would eventually have to become international.

The main indications of acceptable standards in the UK before 1968 were the monographs published in the *British Pharmacopocia*, the first edition of which had appeared in 1864. Prior to this a '*Pharmacopoeia Londiniensis*' was first issued in 1618, and new editions appeared spasmodically until 1851. The equivalent of the *British Pharmacopoeia* for veterinary drugs was the *British Veterinary Codex* which had first been published in 1953. An Addenda and a second edition of the *Veterinary Codex* appeared in 1965, but with the passing of the Medicines Act, it was decided that in future the *British Pharmacopoeia* should cover the requirements of both human and veterinary drugs, although separate volumes would be published.

The first edition of the *British Pharmacopoeia (Veterinary)* appeared in 1977. The *Pharmacopoeia* describes each drug by means of a monograph which covers its chemical structure, the means used to identify it, the requirements for storage, the common types of preparations and the dosages to be used. In addition a note is given on the principal pharmacological actions and uses of the substance.

Medicines Act (1968)

The operation of the Act is controlled by the Medicine Commission which oversees three main committees:

(1) *The Committee on Safety of Medicines* which is responsible for giving advice with respect to safety, quality and efficacy in relation to the human use of any

substance or article covered by the provisions of the Act, and for promoting the collection and investigation of information relating to adverse reactions, so that advice can be given to the Commission on any drug which has shown unacceptable side effects.

(2) *The Veterinary Products Committee* which carries out similar duties to that described under the Committee on Safety of Medicine for all drugs to be used for animal treatment.

(3) *The British Pharmacopoeia Commission* which is responsible for setting chemical standards for all new substances, whether for medical or veterinary use. In addition, it has the duty to update the *British Pharmacopoeia* of medical and veterinary drugs.

The members of the main committees are appointed by the Minister for the Department of Health and Social Security, and the Minister of Agriculture, Fisheries and Food, and are drawn from the academic, clinical and veterinary medicine, pharmaceutical and industrial fields.

As a result of the passing of the Medicines Act a framework has been established which should ensure that all the drugs now used for therapy have a rational basis for their use, that they should be safe for the user, and in the case of animal medications that they will have no deleterious effect on the animal protein which is to be used for human consumption.

Legal control in the USA

Detailed control of medicinal and veterinary drugs began earlier in the USA, and the first legislation came under the general heading of the Food and Drugs Act of 1906. This Act referred to the control and, if necessary, banning of adulterated or misbranded goods from interstate traffic. The Act in practice did not cover all aspects of interstate commerce, and did not prove adequate to deal with medicinal drugs, and in 1927 a separate regulatory agency, The Food, Drug and Insecticide Administration was established. This is more generally known as the FDA (Food and Drug Administration).

Although it proved to be a valuable interstate organization, the FDA did not have sufficient powers to control all aspects of medicinal legislation and it was the unfortunate sequel to a formula change in a sulphanilamide formulation, which led to deaths in patients, that precipitated the tightening of the legislation and brought in the Federal Food, Drug and Cosmetic Act in 1938.

Subsequent amendments to the Act have included regulations controlling veterinary drugs and the Food Additives Amendments of 1958 which contained the 'Delaney Clause' and involved the control and testing of all additives to ensure that there was no evidence that they could induce cancer in man or animals. This requirement has been modified over the years to cover the significance of residues in products of animal origin rather than the relevance of the additive itself. Since 1962 it has also been necessary to prove that any new drug is efficacious, and in 1968 'The Animal Drug Amendments' were published. These consolidated all aspects of the examination of new drugs and also feeds which may contain the drugs. Thus 1968 was a key year in the introduction of drug control in both the UK and the USA.

EEC legislation

Although acceptable drug control legislation throughout the EEC has been slow to be developed, it is likely that EEC legislation will follow closely along the lines defined by the FDA and the Medicines Act of the UK. At present EEC legislation is promulgated in the form of Directives which are sent to all member states so that they can be applied by each individual country. For example, Directives 81/851 and 81/852 were adopted by the European Community in 1981 and applied in the UK in 1983, and they cover all aspects of the control of manufacture, marketing and use of veterinary medicines. 81/851 is concerned with harmonizing the laws of member states in relation to marketing, manufacture and labelling of veterinary products, and 81/852 deals with the analytical, pharmacotoxicological and clinical standards, and protocols which will be followed in the testing of veterinary medicinal products. Directive 70/524, introduced in the late 1970s, covers many feed additives such as coccidiostats and growth promoters which are generally used throughout the Community.

Once all the EEC legislation is effectively harmonized throughout the Community, veterinary medicines will be developed and tested in a way that will be acceptable to countries which are interested in establishing standards for drug usage.

Testing for drug and chemical residues

It has been found in the USA that although much of the food consumed by human beings may contain traces of chemical residues, the tests defined in the legislation have been sufficient to prevent any toxicity problem in humans which can be related to the use of a drug at approved levels in animals (Van Houweling and Norcross 1976). It was estimated in 1974 that approximately 80% of all animals produced for food purposes in the USA receive medication for part, or in some cases, most of their lives. Although similar detailed studies have not been reported in the UK and Europe, it is probable that similar percentages for medication could apply to the farms on which the more intensive systems of management are practised, in the rearing of pigs and poultry. The fact that medication is given to an animal or animals does not of course mean that all animals will receive medication for a prolonged period. A drug may be given to an animal for one to seven days to treat a specific disease condition, or for two to three weeks to cover a period of growth where infection can occur. Whatever the period of treatment, residue studies are of special importance under certain circumstances, such as:

(1) where a drug is to be given in the feed for a period which may include the day prior to slaughter;

(2) where a drug has been given to an animal which has had to go for emergency slaughter; or

(3) where an implant which will remain active for up to 90 days has been placed in an animal, and the date of slaughter cannot be controlled by the licensing agent (government).

Drug usage terminology

In the USA all drugs given to food-producing animals are given a zero permissible residue where this is possible, or alternatively a level of residue which will not exceed FDA tolerances. These are based on the knowledge that there will be no detectable residue at the end of the 'withdrawal time'. Certain terminology is used in legislative documents to describe important areas for drug testing and the definition of those is as follows.

Drug residues

These can include the active principle of a drug and its metabolites and any part of a formulation which might be considered harmful. Information must be supplied to the legislating authority on the results of tests for residues in animal tissues so that a tolerance level can be established for each new drug.

Feed additives

A feed additive is a material which is added to the feed in small quantities to modify or improve some aspects of growth performance.

Target animal

This means the sex and species of animal which will receive the drug.

Acceptable daily intake

This is the level of a chemical which could be ingested daily in the food during the lifetime of a person without causing recognizable toxic harm.

Mutagenic effect

A mutagenic effect may follow the use of a mutagen, a chemical agent which can damage the genetic component of a cell.

Teratogenic effect

A teratogen is a chemical entity which can produce a toxic effect on the growing embryo or foetus and which can result in malformation.

It is usual in all investigations of a new drug to carry out three-generation reproductive studies at an early stage so as to ensure that no damage can be caused to the foetus as a result of the use of the drug.

Drug allergy

A series of hypersensitivity tests are carried out with any new chemicals which are considered to contain an allergic potential.

Margin of safety

Toxicity studies with any new drug always involve establishing the margin of safety for animal use. The margin of acceptable safety varies greatly from drug to drug and a safety factor of 10 is generally considered a satisfactory minimum. When a safety level has been established in the target animal, toxic reactions are seldom seen in the treated animals when the recommended dose is used.

Withdrawal times for veterinary drugs

The establishment of the withdrawal time for a new drug is one of the key decisions that has to be taken before a drug will be approved for marketing. Jackson (1980) defined 'the withdrawal time' as the time required for the residue of toxicologic concern to reach safe concentration as defined by the FDA tolerance level. The withdrawal time intervals vary from drug to drug and in some cases for each species which is to be treated. In the USA existing FDA legislation requires that drug manufacturers submit tissue residue and detection rate studies, and details of the methods of detection of residues on all new animal drug applications so that a withdrawal time can be established.

Sutherland (1969) discussed various methods of establishing safe levels for withholding or withdrawing drugs and the studies depend on establishing first the half-life of a drug in the body.

The study of drug behaviour in the body

Once a drug has been absorbed and has established a concentration in the blood plasma, it is exposed to the various enzymatic and other actions of the body which will ensure its eventual elimination. In some cases, it will be quickly rendered inactive and may be then excreted partly in the intact state and partly as altered molecules.

Metabolism or biotransformation by means of enzymes and chemical changes can either reduce possible toxicity or, in some cases, by selective action such as in a pro-drug, make the drug more effective.

The changes that take place in a drug in the body are classified into two phases of reactions.

Phase 1 reactions

These are usually oxidation, reduction or hydrolysis. The changes that occur can lead to the release of ten or more metabolites of the original drug, which will eventually have to be excreted from the body.

Oxidation is the major phase 1 reaction and is effected by enzymes called oxidases. In the majority of cases the effect of oxidation is to reduce the activity of the chemical, but in some potentially toxic materials such as carbon tetrachloride, the activity is increased and a more toxic metabolite is produced.

The enzymes which are responsible for the *reduction* reactions are known as reductases. Some of them are microsomal (particles formed as a result of biochemical action) in origin, and others are found in the soluble cell fraction. An example of a reduction is the production of sulphanilamide in the body from the chemical prontosil, the first of the important anti-bacterials. Prontosil is an azo dye and the enzyme reductase found in the gut bacteria acts by splitting the azo group.

Prontosil   Sulphanilamide

Metabolism by *hydrolysis* occurs with esters and amides. The enzymes which produce the effect are found in the plasma and the soluble fraction of the cell and they are known as esterases and amidases. An example is the hydrolysis of the insecticide carbaryl by liver enzymes to 1-naphthol.

Phase 2 reactions

The phase 2 reactions usually follow the changes associated with either hydrolysis or oxidation and a drug may be coupled in the liver or kidney with an endogenous substance in a conjugation or synthetic reaction. Various different conjugations can occur but the aim of all is to render the molecule more polar and less lipid-soluble so that it can be readily excreted. The endogenous conjugations are described under a number of headings—glucuronic acid, sulphates, acetylation, amino acids and methylation.

In *glucuronidation*, uridine diphosphate glucuronic acid formed by enzymes in liver cells is able to donate glucuronic acid to a wide variety of substrates.

Sulphate conjugation entails the formation of sulphate esters which can then join with hydroxyl and amino groups. The sulphate donor is 3'-phospho-adenosine-5'-phosphosulphate and the conjugation is catalysed by a sulpho-transferase enzyme. These enzymes are found mainly in the liver, intestinal mucosa and kidney.

Sulphonamides and hydrazines are metabolized by *acetylation*. An enzyme acetyltransferase acts as the catalyst and it is produced in the hepatic reticulo-endothelial cells, in the gastro-intestinal mucosal cells and in some white blood cells.

The commonest *amino acid* used for conjugation is glycine. The reaction involves acylation of the amino group of the amino acid by the carboxylic acid group of the drug to be metabolized.

Amino, hydroxyl and thiol groups in drugs can undergo *methylation*. The reactions are catalysed by methyltransferase enzymes. The methyl donor is S-adenosyl methionine. The methyltransferases are found in the soluble fractions of certain tissues.

The importance of certain factors in the metabolism of drugs

The rate of metabolism of a drug and the efficacy of metabolism can be influenced by a number of factors which can play an important part in the value of drugs in animal therapy. These are briefly described.

Species

Any species difference in the rate of absorption of a drug is of importance in preliminary testing of a drug both for eventual human use and for the use of a drug in a target animal. It is important, therefore, in all preliminary testing to determine the rate of both oral and cutaneous absorption of all new drugs. The examinations should be carried out in a number of species of animals and in particular in the target animal.

Distribution

The distribution of antibiotics and antibacterials may be influenced by plasma binding. If plasma binding is established for a particular drug, the dose of the drug to be used must be adequate to compensate for the proportion which is rendered inactive by binding.

Excretion

Drugs are excreted directly by the gut, kidneys and through the bile into the gut after metabolism in the liver, or through the milk, and via the lungs. The rate of excretion depends on whether a drug passes through the body relatively unchanged or whether it is broken down into a number of metabolites, some of which may persist in the body for a prolonged period. Penicillin, for example, is rapidly absorbed and between 50 and 80% can be recovered from the urine in active form within six hours of dosing. On the other hand, residues of dihydrostreptomycin may be detected in the kidneys for as long as 90 days after a single large injection.

The excretion rate of a drug can, therefore, be of great importance when it is to be used for animal treatment. Excretion is most rapid when a drug or its metabolite is present in an ionized, highly polar form as in this state it will be poorly reabsorbed from the tubular ultrafiltrate.

Withdrawal period, clearance time or detection time

Once the pattern of metabolism and excretion has been established both in the target animal and several laboratory species, it is necessary to establish a safe withdrawal time which will ensure that no toxic or potentially toxic residue is still present in the body of treated animals at the time of slaughter for human consumption. Inevitably the relevance of the established withdrawal period as far as a drug and its metabolites are concerned will depend on the sensitivity of the analytical tests used to reveal the presence of the drug.

It is the aim of the legislator to establish a withdrawal time for all new drugs, so that no residues will be present in the tissues of any animal slaughtered for human consumption. The standard to be set for a drug is often difficult to establish because some workers believe that the concentration of drug in animal will never reach zero. This opinion is based on the fact that elimination curves are plotted logarithmically as declining drug concentrations against time. Some of the graphs would indicate that drug elimination can continue indefinitely.

The fact that the majority of drugs, apart from those used for 'growth promotion' or as 'coccidiostats', are given to animals for short periods of therapy, and that treatment will often occur at a period long removed from the time of slaughter, has to be considered when one is looking at the relevance of drug elimination to the practical use of drugs in animal treatment.

Conclusion

The international legislation for the control of the use of new animal drugs aims to ensure, firstly, that the approved testing programmes will provide the information necessary for the safe use of drugs in the target animal and, secondly, that there will be no unsafe residues left in carcases which are sold for human consumption. In the application of legislation, it is essential that a balance be established between the demands of the law and the eventual economic value of a new drug to the farming community. If the demands of the authorities for information become excessive or are considered unreasonable, and the research and development costs become too expensive for the animal production industry to bear, then the research groups in pharmaceutical companies may be disbanded, and the farmer will be left with relatively ineffective drugs to control outbreaks of serious disease.

The analytical methods developed for testing for drug residues must be practicable for use by government agencies. The major techniques used will depend on radio-labelled drug studies both in laboratory animals and in the animals for which the drug is intended. Residue studies must include all metabolites of the drug produced in the body and tolerance limitations must be established. In addition to laboratory animal examinations the experimental methods described must be suitable for use in field trials, so that withdrawal times can be established for the use of milk from the living animal, and the tissues of other animals before slaughter.

12. The future

Introduction

The twentieth century has seen both veterinary and human medicine develop from being empirical sciences based on 'materia medica' to broadly based sciences which depend for therapeutic advice on the knowledge obtained from pharmacology. Pharmacology is the study of the effect of drugs on the structure and metabolism of normal tissues and this provides the basic information necessary for the evaluation and development of new drugs.

The information which the clinician uses to establish his line of treatment has been acquired both through experimental pharmacological studies on laboratory animals, and applied pharmacology studies which consist in the application of the knowledge acquired from the early experimental studies to the problems of diseased human beings and animals. Many of the original drugs described in the early pharmacopoeias were obtained from plants, and in some cases the active principle had been extracted and concentrated and used for specific purposes. Other material such as fats, oils and resins, and simple minerals such as magnesium, potassium, sodium, copper and iron salts were formulated into suspensions or solutions for general use. In a more specific way, raw liver was used for the control of anaemia. The advances leading to the new drugs of the 1950s, 60s and 70s were achieved by the combined work of the organic chemist, the biochemist and the pharmacologist. This teamwork ensured that all new drugs had a clearly defined structure, and that as much as possible had been learned about the behaviour of a drug in the body before it was used in the clinic or by the veterinary and medical clinician in the field. The future in the search for new opportunities in human and animal medicine is likely to lie in the hands of (a) the geneticist who will indicate the cell manipulations necessary to produce the most effective genes for a specific drug or vaccine, (b) the cell biologist who is aware both of the structure of individual cells and the likely effect of the manipulation of the genes within the cell and (c) the microbiologist who will be responsible for propagating the bacterial cells which will provide the source of many new products.

155

The two main areas of research are likely to be associated with recombinant DNA technology and the use of clones and monoclonal antibodies.

Recombinant DNA

Recombinant DNA or genetic engineering depends on the manipulation of deoxyribonucleic acid (DNA) which carries the hereditary information in a cell. It is possible to insert into the DNA of a host cell (most frequently a non-pathogenic bacterium), a length of DNA which can carry the genetic instructions coding for a possible medicinal product that is difficult to synthesize by normal chemical means, such as insulin. The DNA may be cut into lengths and inserted into the bacterial cell and then bound to a matrix within the cell. This work has become possible only by the use of the electron microscope which has so enlarged bacteria and viruses to the viewer that it is possible to use probes to open a cell and insert the appropriate section of DNA at a specific site in the cell.

Clones

A clone of cells consists of the progeny of a single parental cell and the cells are produced by repeated mitotic cell divisions, usually by asexual multiplication in bacteria or viruses. The aim of cloning is to achieve such replication, so that each cell is identical. Most of this work to date has been carried out using plants, bacteria and viruses.

It is also now possible using fertilized animal eggs to divide the egg into two equal parts and then return the identical clones into the uterus and so produce a pair of identical twins.

The use of recombinant DNA and clones

It is likely that these two lines of research will, in the veterinary field, lead to:
(1) new improved vaccines for the prevention of animal disease;
(2) more specific growth promoters;
(3) the more economical development of antibiotics and possibly new antibiotics;
(4) new therapeutic agents;
(5) nutritional materials which are more economical than many naturally available supplements such as amino acids and vitamins;
(6) diagnostic tools for the definition of specific diseases in a farm unit.

Vaccines

It has always been the aim of vaccine developers to refine vaccine production so that only the key antigens are present in the vaccine. Many viruses and bacteria contain, in addition to antigens, toxic elements and other substances which play no part in stimulating an immune response in the host. The aim, therefore, would be, by genetic engineering, to use for vaccine production viral or bacterial cells which contain only the specific genes for the protein molecules which stimulate immunity, and to remove any genes which are responsible for toxic reactions in any host which may receive them. It is possible by the use of genetic engineering to influence the gene content of bacteria and viruses and this can be achieved in a variety of ways.

(1) It is possible to remove the essential genes of a pathogenic bacterium or virus and develop attenuated strains which can be safely used in the animal host.

(2) The genes responsible for coding the toxic effect of a pathogen can be identified and removed from a cell so that the vaccine produced contains only non-pathogenic immunogens.

(3) It is possible to clone cells to express the surface antigens in numbers which will provide a safe vaccine.

There are a number of vaccines both in the animal and human fields which could be improved in this way. In foot-and-mouth disease of cattle and pigs it might be possible to develop a vaccine which contains genes for proteins found in all the different virus strains of the disease, and in a similar way a human influenza vaccine might be produced which would contain a multiplicity of known virus strains.

Other diseases such as the tropical diseases spread by ticks and tsetse flies which are now poorly controlled by the use of chemotherapeutic agents might be controlled by vaccines which contain the essential genes of the infecting protozoa developed within a non-pathogenic bacterium.

Growth promoters

Growth promoters in the future may be developed by genetic engineering to provide animal food materials which can stimulate improved growth at a cost lower than that required when an animal obtains the same materials from expensive cereals. L-Tryptophan is an example of an amino acid which is likely to be produced in this way.

A growth promoter known as bovine growth hormone (BGH) has involved the use of recombinant DNA technology and is being investigated for its value in stimulating increased milk production in dairy cattle (Bines *et al*. 1980). A consistent increase in milk production follows daily administration of this hormone. It is suggested (Peel *et al*. 1983) that the growth hormone achieves its effect by increasing the synthesis of nucleic acids and protein in many tissues. The increased mammary gland synthesis of RNA could be followed by the synthesis of a number of key enzymes which could then enhance the synthesis of all milk components.

Other hormones are likely to be developed which by increasing the synthesis of nucleic acids will accelerate the general growth rate.

Development of more economic antibiotics

The selection of more effective strains for the production of antibiotics from fungal moulds or bacterial sources is already practised, but it seems likely that the cloning of specific genes or recombinant DNA technology will increase the yields of antibiotic from existing sources. It might also be possible by means of the fusion of active DNA from different antibiotic-producing organisms to generate new antibiotics.

New therapeutic agents

The progress that has already been made in the development of a new insulin product by genetic engineering suggests that future opportunities may lie in the production of antivirals and other agents which cannot be simply developed either by the normal processes of fermentation growth, as in penicillin, or by synthesis using the normal processes of organic chemistry.

The likely new products lie in the following fields:
(1) hormones and growth promoters;
(2) antivirals and antiprotozoal and antihelminth products;
(3) monoclonal antibodies, which will be of particular value in assisting in the identification of specific strains of antigens. They can also be used to protect young animals during the first 24 hours of life against lethal pathogens.

Nutritional materials

It is already possible to produce amino acids such as lysine by the use of recombinant DNA using the organisms *Corynebacterium* or *Brevibacterium*. The cost of production would have to be lower than using, for example, soya bean as a key source of lysine.

Genetic engineering can be used to improve the yield of single-cell protein so that the most genetically effective cells can be used on the substrate. Various substrates are used and others are under investigation so that the most effective growth medium can be used for the cells. Materials which are being used or tested include waste starch, wood pulp, methane and methanol. The economic success of single-cell protein is very closely related to the yield that can be obtained from the organism used.

Diagnostic tools

Synthetic DNA probes can be used to identify pathogens, such as bacteria or viruses, which have been recovered from diseased animals. To produce the diagnostic agent, the cell which is to be identified is disrupted and the DNA is isolated. The DNA is separated into single strands which are fixed to a matrix. Labelled single-stranded DNA probes of known structure are added and allowed to hybridize with the DNA which is fixed to the matrix. Unhybridized probes are washed off and the hybridized DNA probe is identified.

All these possible areas for development are being investigated, but each in its different way will offer problems which will have to be solved before any product can be confidently marketed. In the case of improving foot-and-mouth vaccines, for instance, an antigenic sub-unit of foot-and-mouth disease vaccine can be produced in bacteria in large quantities. However, there are still problems related to finding the best method of presenting the antigen to the host so that a good immune response is stimulated.

Control and regulation of the new technology

The new technology, which will require legislation additional to that already applied to new medicines, will depend for its success on an acceptance by the authorities that the techniques applied are not frightening, but can lead to the production of new drugs which will improve disease control methods and also assist in the production of food for the world population. There are three main aspects of the likely regulations:

(1) regulation of the process, i.e. the discovery, the development and manufacturing techniques;

(2) regulation of the end product, i.e. therapeutic use or use as a diagnostic agent;

(3) regulations which may be necessary to protect the environment.

Regulations for control of the new techniques are being developed in the UK and Europe, the USA and by the World Health Organization. The eventual acceptance and success of new products based on the biotechnology will depend on the ability of government assessors to appreciate the likely benefits of a new concept, and also on their ability to take the decisions which will allow a step forward in gene manipulation to take place.

Finally the end user, the farmer and the customer, must be made aware in a simple manner of the benefits of the new development and also be assured that there are no long-term, unacceptable risks.

References and further reading

Chapter 1

Schwabe, C. W., 1978, *Cattle, Priests and Progress in Medicine* (University of Minnesota Press).

Toynbee, J. M. C., 1973, *Animals in Roman Life and Art* (London: Thames & Hudson).

Chapter 2

Andrewes, C. H. and Walton, J. R., 1977, *Viral and bacterial zoonoses* (London: Baillière Tindall).

Baxter, S. H., Baxter, M. R. and MacCormack, J. A., 1983, *Farm Animal Housing and Welfare* (Boston and The Hague: Martinus Nijhoff).

Dyer, I. A. and O'Mary, C. C., 1977, *The Feed Lot* (Philadelphia: Lea and Febiger).

Hartley, C. L. and Richmond, M. H., 1975, 'Antibiotic resistance and the survival of *E. coli* in the alimentary tract', *Br. Med. J.*, **4**, 71.

Jensen, R. and Mackey, D. R., 1971, *Diseases of Feed-lot Cattle* (Philadelphia: Lea and Febiger).

Wilson, G., 1974, 'The use of epidemiology in animal disease', *Vet. J.*, **130**, 207.

Chapter 3

Baxter, S. H., 1969, *Scottish Farm Buildings Investigation Unit Report No. 4.*

Brander, G. C. and Ellis, P. R., 1977, *The Control of Disease* (London: Baillière Tindall).

Christie, A. B., 1980, *Infectious diseases: Epidemiology and Clinical Practice*, 3rd edition (Edinburgh: Churchill Livingstone).

Freeman, A. M., Haverman, R. H. and Kneese, A. V., 1973, *The Economics of Environmental Policy* (New York: Wiley).

Muirhead, M. R., 1983, 'Pig Housing and Environment', *Vet. Rec.*, Dec. 17, pp. 587–93.

Rossiter, P. B., Jessett, D. M., Wafula, J. S., Karstadl, C. S., Taylor, W. P., Rowe, L., Nyange, J. C., Otarum Mumbala, M., Scott, G. R., 1983, 'Re-emergence of rinderpest as a threat in East Africa since 1979', *Vet. Rec.*, **113** (20), 459–61.

Schwabe, C. W., Rieman, H. R. and Franti, C. E., 1977, *Epidemiology in Veterinary Practice* (Philadelphia: Lea and Febiger).

Chapter 4

Dewey, D. W., Lee, H. J. and Marston, H. R., 1958, 'Provision of cobalt to ruminants by means of heavy pellets', *Nature*, **181**, 1367–71.

Doll, R., 1983, 'The prospects for prevention', *B.M.J.*, **286**, 445.

Monkhouse, D. C., 1978, *Animal Health Products Design and Evaluation* (Washington D.C.: American Pharmaceutical Association).

The Value of Preventive Medicine, 1985, Ciba Foundation Symposium Pitman Publishing.

Chapter 5

Batchelor, F. R., Doyle, F. P., Naylor, J. H. and Rolinson, G. N., 1959, *Nature*, **183**, 257.

Brander, G. C., Pugh, P. M. and Bywater, R. J., 1982, *Veterinary Applied Pharmacology and Therapeutics* (London: Baillière Tindall).

Chain, E., Florey, H. W., Gardner, A. D., Heatley, N. G., Jennings, M. A., Orr-Ewing, J. and Sanders, A. G., 1940, 'Penicillin as a chemotherapeutic agent', *Lancet*, 24 August.

Fleming, A., 1929, *Br. J. Exp. Path.*, **10**, 226.

Garrod, L. P., 1970, 'Conquest of Microbic Disease by Drugs', *British Medicine Bulletin*, **26** (3), 187.

Garrod, L. P., Lambert, H. P. and O'Grady, F., 1981, *Antibiotics and Chemotherapy* (Edinburgh: Churchill Livingstone).

Hitchings, G. H., 1961, 'A biochemical approach to chemotherapy', *Trans. N.Y. Acad. Sci.*, **23**, 700–8.

Newton, G. G. F. and Abraham, E. P., 1956, 'Isolation of cephalosporin C – penicillin-like antibiotic', *Biochem. J.*, **62**, 651–8.

Chapter 6

Anthelmintics for Cattle and Sheep, 1982, A.D.A.S. Booklet 2412, 26pp.

Armour, J. and Bogan, J., 1982, 'Anthelmintics for ruminants', *British Vet. J.*, **138**, 371–82.

Pritchard, R. K., 1978, *Epidemiology and Control of Gastro-intestinal Parasites of Sheep* (Canberra: C.S.I.R.O.).

Pritchard, R. K., Steel, J. W., Lacey, E. and Hennessy, D. R., 1985, Pharmacokinetics of ivermectin in sheep following intravenous, intra-abomasal, and intraruminal administration', *J. Vet. Pharmacol. Therapeutics* (8 January 1985).

Soulsby, E. J. L., 1982, *Helminths, Arthropods and Protozoa of Domesticated Animals* (London: Baillière Tindall).

Chapter 7

Beeman, R. W., 1982, *Ann. Rev. Entomol.*, **27**, 253–81.

Brown, A. W. and Pal, R., 1971, *Insecticide Resistance in Arthropods* (Monograph No. 38) (Geneva: WHO).

Campbell, W. C. and Rev, R. S. (editors), 1985, *Chemotherapy of Parasitic Diseases* (New York: Plenum Press).
Campbell, W. C., Fisher, M. H., Stapley, E. O., Albers-Schönberg, G. and Jacob, T. A., 1983, *Science*, **221**, No. 4613.
Corbett, J. R., Wright, K. and Baille, A. C., 1983, *The Biochemical Mode of Action of Pesticides* (London: Academic Press).
Elliott, M., 1973, 'A photostable pyrethroid', *Nature*, **246**, 169–70
Kuhr, R. J. and Dorough, H. W., 1976, *Carbamate Insecticides; Chemistry, Biochemistry and Toxicology* (Cleveland, OH: CRC Press).
Leahey, J. P. (ed), 1985, *The Pyrethroid Insecticides* (London: Taylor & Francis).
Lund, A. E., Hollingworth, W. and Murdock, L. L., 1979, In *Advances in Pesticide Science*, edited by H. Geissbühler, Part 3 (Oxford: Pergamon Press), pp. 465–9.
Narahashi, T., 1962, *J. Cell. Comp. Physiol.*, **59**, 61–5.
Uchida, M., Fujita, T., Kurihara, N. and Nakajima, M., 1978, In *Pesticide and Venom Neurotoxicity*, edited by D. L. Shankland, R. M. Hollingworth and T. Smyth Jr. (New York: Plenum Press), pp. 133–51.

Chapter 8

Aliu, Y. O., Davis, R. H., Camp, B. J. and Kuttler, K. L., 1977, *Am. J. Vet. Res.*, **38**, 2001.
Cruthers, L. R. and Szanto, J., 1980, In *Veterinary Medicine*, edited by A. T. Phillipson, L. W. Hall and W. R. Pritchard (London: William Heinemann).
Klein, R. A., 1980, *Principles in the Chemotherapy of Protozoan Disease* (London: Heinemann).
McDougall, L. R. and Long, P. L., 1984, *Handbook of Poultry Parasitology* (New York: Praeger Scientific).
Molyneux, D. H. and Ashford, R. W., 1983, *The Biology of Trypanosoma and Leishmania, Parasites of Man and Domestic Animals* (London: Taylor & Francis).
Newton, B. A., 1970, 'Chemotherapeutic compounds affecting DNA structure and function', *Adv. Pharm. Chemotherap.*, **8**, 149–84.
Roby, T. O., Simpson, J. E. and Amerault, T. E., 1978, *Am. J. Vet. Res.*, **39**, 1115.
Soulsby, E. J. L., 1982, *Helminths, Arthropods and Protozoa of Domesticated Animals* (London: Baillière Tindall).
Williamson, J., 1970, 'Review of chemotherapeutic and chemoprophylactic agents', in *The African Trypanosomiases*, edited by H. W. Mulligan and W. H. Potts (London: Allen & Unwin), pp. 125–221.

Chapter 9

Coates, M. E., Davies, M. K., Kon, S. K., 1955, 'The effect of antibiotics on the intestine of the chick', *Brit. J. Nutrit.*, **9**, 110.
Committee to study the human health effects of sub-therapeutic antibiotic use in animals, 1980 (National Academy of Sciences).
Heitzman, R. J., 1976, in *Anabolic Agents in Animal Production*, edited by H. C. Lu and J. Rendel, Environmental Quality and Safety Suppl. V p. 89.
Heitzman, R. J., 1978, *Nutrition Conference for Feed manufacturers No. 13. Recent advances in animal nutrition*, edited by W. Haresign and D. Lewis (London: Butterworth), p. 133.

Roche, J. F. and O'Callaghan, D., 1984, *Manipulation of Growth in Farm Animals.* (The Hague: Martinus Nijhoff).

Swann, M. M., 1968, *Report of the Joint Committee on the Use of Antibiotics in Animal Husbandry and Veterinary Medicine* (London: HMSO).

Visek, W. J., 1978, 'The mode of growth promotion by antibiotics', *J. Animal Sci.*, **46**, 5.

Walton, J. R., 1983, 'Antibiotics, animals, meat and milk', *Zbl. Vet. Med.* A, **30**, 81–92. (Journal of Vet. Medicine series A.)

Chapter 11

Booth, N. H. and McDonald, L. E., 1982, *Veterinary, Pharmacology and Therapeutics* (Ames, USA: The Iowa State University Press).

Brander, G. C., Pugh, D. M. and Bywater, R. J., 1982, *Veterinary Applied Pharmacology and Therapeutics* (London: Baillière Tindall).

Brinley Morgan, W. J., 1983, 'Legislation covering the licensing of veterinary medicines in the United Kingdom', *Vet. Rec.*, **113** (14), 310.

Jackson, B. A., 1980, *J. Am. Vet. Med. Assoc.*, **176**, 1141.

Medicines Act (1968) HMSO.

Nelson, N. *et al.*, 1970, Food and Drug Administration Advisory Committee on Protocols for Safety Evaluations, *Toxicol. Appl. Pharmacol.*, **16**, 264–96.

Shillam, K. W. G., 1974, *J. Sci. Food Agric.*, **25**, 227.

Staff Medicines Unit (CVL), 1983, EEC Veterinary Directives, *Vet. Rec.* **113** (14), 313.

Sutherland, G. L., 1969, *Proceedings of a Symposium on the Use of Drugs in Animal Feeds* No. 1679, p. 244 (Washington D.C.: National Academy of Sciences).

Timbrell, J. A., 1982, *Principles of Biochemical Toxicology* (London: Taylor & Francis).

Van Houweling, J. D. and Norcross, M. A., 1976, *Vet. Hum. Toxicology*, **18**, 130.

Chapter 12

Allen, C. E., 1983, 'New horizons in animal agriculture: future challenges for agricultural scientists', *Animal Sci.*, **57**, Supplement 2, 16–27.

Association of Veterinarians in Industry, *New Biotechnology for Animal Health and Production (1983) Symposium* (The Librarian, Royal College of Veterinary Surgeons, Wellcome Library, London).

Bines, J. A., Hart, I. C. and Morant, S. V., 1980, *Br. J. Nutrition*, **43**, 179–88.

Gibson, R., 1982, 'Genetic manipulation, principles and practices', *Biologist*, **29**, 191–7.

Moore, D. M., 1983, Introduction of a vaccine for foot and mouth disease through gene cloning. Beltsville Symposia in agricultural research. Genetic engineering in agriculture, *Recombinant Technology, May 1982* (Montclair: Allanheld, Osmun), pp. 132–42.

Old, R. W. and Primrose, S. B., 1981, *Principles of Gene Manipulation – an Introduction to Genetic Engineering*, Studies in Microbiology, Vol. 2 (Oxford: Blackwell Scientific).

Peel, C. J. Frank, T. J., Bauman, D. E. and Gorewin, R. C., 1983, *J. Dairy Sci.*, **66**, 776–82.

Index

165